Auricular Acupuncture Therapy

Written by Xiao Fei Wei Lushuang
Transtated by Xiao Fei Jing Zhen

Shandong Science and Technology Press

First Edition 1996
ISBN 7-5331-1835-9

Auricular Acupuncture Therapy

Written by Xiao Fei Wei Lushuang
Translated by Xiao Fei Jing Zhen
Editor in charge Li Yu

Published by Shandong Science and Technology Press
16 Yuhan Road, Jinan, China 250002
Printed by Shandong Lai Wu Printing House
Distributed by China International Book Trading Corporation
35 Chegongzhuang Xilu, Beijing 100044, China
P.O. Box 399, Beijing, China
Printed in the People's Republic of China

Praface

This book is one volume of *The Series of Traditional Chinese Medicine for Foreign Readers.*

Rarely, a medical therapy has been spreading so quickly and widely and liked so much by both medical workers and patients as auricular acupuncture therapy. Why is it so appealling? The answer is that this therapy is convenient to use, easy to study and effective against diseases. It is so convenient that it can be applied even without any instruments; it is so easy to study that one may apply this therapy right after reading it, and it is so effective that therapeutic effectiveness is often present soon after treatment. Besides, auricular acupuncture produces little side effects. To introduce the most present achievements to the world outside China and further improve the applications of auricular acupuncture, we wrote this book on the basis of collection of all data relevant and available and our experience.

The contents of this book mainly include anatomy of the auricle, location, function and indication of auricular points, various methods of auricular acupuncture therapy, auricular diagnosis, and auricular treatment. On the bases of introduction to the fundamental knowledge of auricular acupuncture, emphasis is put to the practical knowledge or clinical application. For compiling this book, we made much efforts in the following aspects:

1. Diseases selected carefully: Any therapy has its indications, so does the auricular acupuncture therapy. According to the author's experience, auricular acupuncture may be highly effective for some diseases but not for all

diseases. Therefore, only those that are sensitive to auricular acupuncture are selected. A total of 40 diseases were discussed.

2. Methods explained in detail: In order to suit the reader'use, different treatment methods of auricular acupuncture are explained in detail, such as needling, intradermal-needle-embedding, seed-pressing, drug injection, magnetic therapy and bleeding therapy. Furthermore, according to the features of each disease, we introduced the suitable methods so that the readers may select one of these for their convenience.

3. Words and illustration being combined: To facilitate clinical practice, each disease is attached an illustration marked with all auricular points being used. Therefore, the reader can perform treatment without reviewing the previous knowledge.

This book is suitable for persons who are interested in auricular acupuncture therapy, especially the clinicians.

Xiao Fei
Affiliated Hospital of Shandong
University of TCM
Jinan
P. R. China

Contents

Introduction

Ⅰ. Brief History of Auricular Acupuncture

Auricular acupuncture is an unique therapeutic method in which the auricle is used to diagnose and treat diseases. Since puncture has been the principal stimulating method, it is still habitually called auricular acupuncture therapy though numbers of methods have been developed up to now, such as seed-pressing, intradermal-needle-embedding and laser irradiation.

Auricular acupuncture has a considerable long history. In China, it may date back to the Warring State period (400－500 B. C.). However, the knowledge of auricular acupuncture had been scattered and had not been paid much attention to before P. R. China was founded in 1949. It is in the 1950's that auricular acupuncture was put forwards and advocated as a relatively independent unique therapeutic method.

In the Warring State period, *Zu Bi Shi Yi Mai Jiu Jing* (Moxibustion Classic and Eleven Channels of Foot-Hand) and *Yin Yang Shi Yi Mai Jiu Jing* (Moxibustion Classic and Eleven Channels of Yin-Yang) recorded auricular Meridians which associates with the arm, eye, cheek and throat, indicating that the auricle was used to diagnose and treat diseases that times. *Nei Jing* (Internal Classic), slightly later than the above works, recorded the relationship between the ear and Zang-Fu organs and Meridians, providing a theoretical basis for the application of auricular acupuncture. Besides, *Nei Jing* (Internal Classic) also records some concrete applications of the auricle in diagnosing and treating diseases. For example, the chapter *Wu Xie* (Five Pathogenic Factors) of *Ling Shu* (Miraculous Pivot) says that pathogenic factors stayed in the Liver may cause hypochondriac pain and convulsion, which can be treated at blue veins of the auricle. The chapter *Liao Ci* (Controlateral Puncturing) of *Su Wen* (Plain Questions) says that *Shi Jue* (Corpse-Like Syncope) can be treated by blowing the two ears with a bamboo pipe.

In the Jin Dynasty, *Zhou Hou Bei Ji Fang* (A Handbook of Prescription for Emergency) written by Ge Hong recorded the clinical application of auricular therapy. For example, it says that for sudden loss of consciousness, quick response may be present following pouring mashed Chinese chives into the ear and blowing *Zao Jiao* (Spine Gleditsian) into the nose.

In the Tang Dynasty, *Qian Jin Yao Fang* (Thousand Ducat Prescriptions)and *Qian Jin Yi Fang* (Supplemental Wings to the Thousand Ducat Prescriptions) written by Sun Simiao recorded auricular diagnostic method and the location, indication and treatment method of two auricular points, Er Zhong and Er Wei.

In the Ming Dynasty, *Zhen Jiu Da Cheng* (Great Compendium of Acupuncture and Moxibustion) written by Yang Jizhou recorded the location, method for locating, treatment method and indications of Er Jian (Ear Apex). It states that moxibustion at Er Jian can cure nebula while at Er Men can cure dental caries.

In the Qing Dynasty, *Li Zheng An Mo Yao Shu* (Revised Important Techniques of Massage) written by Zhang Zhenyun recorded the method of observing the ear. This book has a chapter of *Cha Er*

(Observing the Ear) specially dealing with how to diagnose disease with the ear. There is also an auricular point illustration of the posterior surface of the auricle recorded, on which the distribuation of the five Zang organs are described. This may be the first illustration of auricular points in the world.

The rapid development of auricular acupuncture started from the late 1950s. Since then on, auricular acupuncture has attracted more and more attention. In China, a report on acute tonsillitis successfully treated with auricular acupuncture was published in 1956, which evoked medical workers' interesting. At the same time, P. Nogier, M. D., a Frenchman who had studied acupuncture in China, published a paper in Germany, in which he pointed out the close relation between the auricle and the internal organs and proposed an "inverted-fetus like" auricular point illustration on the basis of tender spots found in his clinical practice. This point illustration was soon briefly introduced by Xiao Lin in Shanghai Journal of Traditional Chinese Medicine, which greatly inspired TCM doctors and aroused their ferve to research this unique therapy. In 1959, Xu Zoulin reported 225 cases treated with auricular acupuncture and proposed 15 auricular stimulating points. By the middle 1960s, the number of Chinese auricular points had reached 100.

In the 1970s, the development of auricular acupuncture reached its first peak. According to statistics, the number of auricular points increased up to 700 and the diseases reported to be effectively treated with auricular acupuncture was as many as 150. Auricular diagnosis was also made a great progress in this period. Besides, A number of monographic works were published, such as *Er Zhen Liao Fa* (Auricular Therapy) written by medical workers in the Animal Institute of China Academy of Science and *Er Zhen* (Auricular Acupuncture) written by Wang Zhong. In this period, auricular acupuncture also quickly spreaded in France, Germany, Japan, the USA, etc.

In the 1980s, the standardization of auricular acupuncture and experimental study on its therapeutic mechanism were emphasized. In the 1970s, the nomenclature and location of auricular points were somewhat in disorder, which hampered the development and academic exchange of auricular therapy. To meet the rapid development of auricular acupuncture, a great number of auricular acupuncture institutes were founded. For example, the Auricular Acupuncture Group of All-China Acupuncture and Moxibustion Association and Yunnan Institute of Auricular Acupuncture were established in the meeting of China Conference of Acupuncture and Moxibustion Techniques held in 1982. In 1987, the WHO Regional office for the Western Pacific held the Third WHO Regional Working Group Meeting on the Standardization of Acupuncture Nomenclature in Seoul. At this meeting, the nomenclature and location of auricular points were standardized on the basis of the plan proposed by the China Association of Acupuncture and Moxibustion, which terminates the disorder state of the development of auricular acupuncture and makes it canonical and international.

Ⅱ. The Theoretical Basis of Auricular Acupuncture

Traditional Chinese Medicinal theory of Zang-Fu organs and Meridians is the principal theoretical basis of auricular acupuncture. In addition, the extensive relation between the auricle and the nervous system and theory of Embryo Complete Information of Wholistic Organ (ECIWO), etc. also sever as the theoretical basis.

1. The theory of Traditional Chinese Medicine

In Traditional Chinese Medicine (TCM), the auricle is considered to be closely related with Meridians and Zang-Fu organs.

(1) Relations between the auricle and Zang-Fu organs

Explanation of the mechanism of using auricular points to treat diseases of the whole body can date back to *Nei Jing* (Internal Classic). The book states that the ear is very closely related to Meridians. The chapter *Xie Qi Zang Fu Bing Xing Pian* (Manifestations of Pathogenic Factors and Zang-Fu Organs) of *Ling Shu* (Miraculous Pivot) says that Blood and Qi in the twelve Channels and three hundred and sixty-five Collaterals run upwards to the face and then enter the orifices... the rest of the Qi enters the ear to support hearing ability. The chapter *Jing Mai* (Meridians) of *Ling Shu*(Miraculous Pivot) describes the distribution of six Yang Channels in the ear:

One branch of the Small Intestine Channel of Hand-Taiyang enters the ear.

One branch of the Sanjiao Channel of Hand-Shaoyang originates behind the ear, runs upwards along the posterior border of the ear and enters the superior aspect of the ear. Another branch arises from the retro-auricular region, enters the ear, and then emerges in front of the ear.

One branch of the Gallbladder Channel of Foot-Shaoyang runs from the retro-auricular region to the ear and then emerges in front of the ear.

The Divergent Channel of Hand-Yangming enters the ear and joins the Zong Jing (Assembled Channel).

The Stomach Channel of Foot-Yangming ascends to the preauricular region.

One branch of the Bladder Channel of Foot-Taiyang splits off the main trunk, runs from the vertex of the head, and descends to the upper aspect of the auricle.

Although the six Yin Channels do not enter the ear or reach its surroundings directly, they associate with the ear via their Divergent Channels (Jing Bie) which connect the Yang Channels. Therefore, all the Twelve Regular Channels associate the ear either directly or indirectly. Hence the chapter *Kou Wen* (Question) of *Ling Shu* (Miraculous Pivot) says that the ear is the assembled place of Channels.

The relation between the ear and Meridians has also been confirmed by Channel transmission which is induced by stimulating auricular points. The Teaching and Researching Group of Acupuncture Anesthesia, Guangzhou University of Traditional Chinese Medicine, conducted a trial on stimulating auricular points to elicit Channel transmission. Among 104 times of examination, Channel transmission was elicited in 90 (accounting for 86.5%), indicating a specific relationship between the stimulated point and or Channels and Channel transmission.

(2) Relations between the auricle and Zang-Fu organs

There are physiological relations between the auricle and Zang-Fu organs. Among the five Zang organs, the Kidney is the organ most closely related with the ear, second to which are the Heart and the Lung. The chapter *Mai Du* (Measurement of Meridians) of *Ling Shu* (Miraculous Pivot)states that the Kidney Qi connects with the ear, therefore, a sound Kidney is the basis of the hearing function of the ear. The chapter *Jin Gui Zhen Yan Lun* (Maxim of Golden Chamber) of *Su Wen* (Plain Questions) says that the ear connects with the Heart. *Si Shi Nan* (The Fortieth Difficulty) of *Nan Jing* (Classic of Difficulties) states that the Lung controls voice and enables the ear to hear. As early as in 1888, Zhang Zhenjun collected the experience recorded in ancient medical works and proposed a doctrine of distribution of five Zang organs on the auricle.

Clinical observation and experimental study have confirmed that a specific relation exists between the ear and the five Zang organs. A trial on patients suffering from acute myocardial infarction displayed that the locus of Heart (MA—IC) presented congestive flush in 81.7% of the subjects and the locus of Small Intestine (MA—SC2) in 73.3% of the subjects.

2. The theory of Neurography

The auricle is richly supplied with nerves. Principal nerves include the great auricular nerve and lesser occipital nerve, which derive from the plexus of the spinal nerve, the auriculotemporal nerve, which derives from the cranial nerve, and branches from the facial nerve, glossopharyngeal nerve, vagus nerve and sympathetic nerve. Besides, the auricular skin contains a variety of neuroreceptors, such as free sensory nerve endings, follicular sensory nerve endings and corpuscula lamellosa. In the tendon and muscle of the auricle, there are plexiform sensory nerve endings both simple and complex, Golgi tendon organs, Ruffini's nerve endings and muscular spindles. Therefore, the auricular points are highly sensitive to various stimuli.

3. The theory of Embryo Complete Information of Wholistic Organ (ECIWO)

In 1973, Professor Zhang Yingqing proposed ECIWO, which offers a new theoretical basis for application of auricular therapy. ECIWO holds that any relatively independent part of the body, such as each of the Zang-Fu organs, four limbs, all bones, the ear, the nose, the mouth, etc., contains information of the whole organism or is the miniature of it. According to the theory, the ear, as a comparatively independent part of the body, contains life information corresponding to the whole body. Therefore, disorders of the body can reflect themselves on the auricle, and observing and analyzing those positive reactions can help make diagnosis and stimulating specific points of the auricle can treat corresponding diseases.

Ⅲ. The Characteristics of Auricular Acupuncture

1. **Regulating the body function without disturbing the homeostasis**

The therapeutic mechanism of auricular acupuncture is regularity. It inhibits what is hyperactive while promotes what is hypoactive, producing little influence on healthy tissues and organs. For example, stimulating specific points can lower blood pressure in patients with hypertension but elevate it in patients with hypotension. As soon as the blood pressure return to normal level, auricular acupuncture produces action on it. In other words, the therapy will not lower hypertension to abnormally low level and elevate hypotension to abnormally high level.

Different from pharmacotherapy, auricular acupuncture treats and prevents diseases by stimulating auricular points to arouse the body's potential power via the relation of life information between the auricle and the body. It is therefore will not disturb the homeostasis of the organism, which is what the modern medicine has seeking all the time.

2. Wide indications and quick response

Theoretically, auricular acupuncture is effective for treating any disease. The present clinical data shows that as many as 300 kinds of diseases have been reported to be effectively treated with auricular acupuncture, of which about 100 are fairly good response to it. These involve diseases of a variety of systems or clinical departments, such as the internal disease, the surgical disease, the paediatric disease, the ophthalmological disease, the ear, nose and throat diseases, and the dental disease. Generally, auricular acupuncture produces satisfactory therapeutic effectiveness for pain syndromes and functional disorders. It also demonstrates an unique advantages in cessation of smoking or drug, and weight reduction.

Auricular acupuncture often produces quick response. For example, response is often noticed several minutes after start of the treatment in treating headache, toothache, lumbago and stomachache, and after one to two treatments in treating insomnia and for cessation of smoking and weight reduction.

3. Assisting diagnose

Although auricular acupuncture is mainly used to treat and prevent diseases, it is also useful for assisting diagnosis. Being simple and convenient, auricular diagnosis demonstrates a bright future. The present considerable data show that it is of great value to the diagnosis of tumor, hepatitis and ischemic heart disease.

Auricular Points

I . Anatomical Areas of the Auricle

1. Anatomical areas of the anterior auricular surface

In the anterior surface of the auricle, there are four prominences, three depressions, four notches and one ear lobe (Fig. 2—1).

Helix: The curling rim of the most lateral border of the auricle, consisting of the root of the helix, the tubercle of the helix and the end of the helix. The root of the helix or the helix crus refers to the transverse ridge of the helix continuing backwards into the ear cavity; the helix tubercle the small tubercle at the lateral-superior aspect of the helix; and the end of the helix the lowest border of the helix connecting with the ear lobe.

Antihelix: At the medial aspect of the helix, a "Y" form protruding curving ridge parallel to the helix. It is divided into three parts, superior antihelix crus, inferior helix crus and body of antihelix. The superior antihelix crus refers to the upper branch of the antihelix, the inferior antihelix crus the lower branch of the antihelix, and the body of the antihelix the lower part of the antihelix.

Tragus: A curved flap in front of the auricle. There are two obvious prominences in the tragus: the upper apex of the tragus and the lower apex of the tragus.

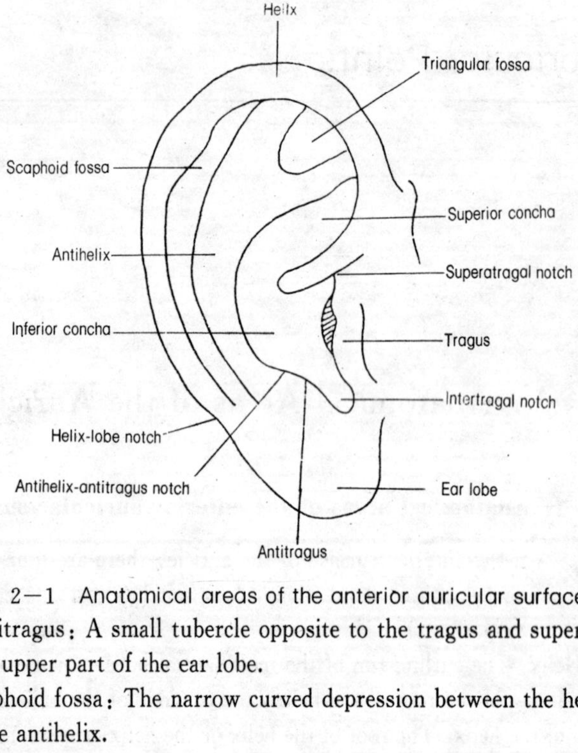

Fig. 2—1 Anatomical areas of the anterior auricular surface

Antitragus: A small tubercle opposite to the tragus and superior to the upper part of the ear lobe.

Scaphoid fossa: The narrow curved depression between the helix and the antihelix.

Triangular fossa: The triangular depression between the two crura of the antihelix.

Concha: The depression encircled by the antitragus, the curving part of the antihelix and the inferior antihelix crus. It consists of two parts, superior concha and inferior concha. The superior concha or cymba conchae refers to the cavum superior to the helix crus while the inferior concha or cavum conchae refers to the cavum inferior to the helix crus.

Ear lobe: The lowest part of the auricle without cartilage.

Supratragal notch: The depression between the upper border of the tragus and the helix crus.

Intertragal notch: The depression between the tragus and the antitragus.

Antihelix-antitragus notch: The depression between the antitragus and the antihelix.

Helix-lobe notch: The depression between the helix and posterior border of the ear lobe.

2. Anatomical areas of the posterior auricular surface

There are three flat areas, five grooves and four prominences in the posterior surface of the auricle (Fig. 2—2).

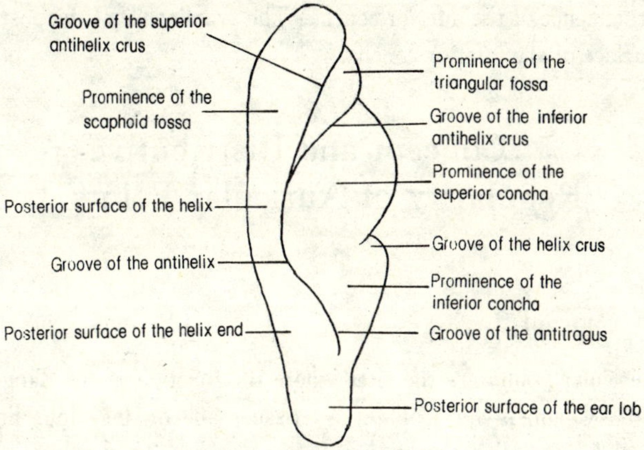

Fig. 2—2 Anatomical areas of the posterior auricular surface

Posterior surface of the helix: Lateral aspect of the helix. Since the helix curves forwards, the aspect faces ahead.

Posterior surface of the helix end: The flat area between the posterior surfaces of the scaphoid fossa and the ear lobe.

Posterior surface of the ear lobe: The flat area of the posterior surface of the ear lobe.

Groove of the antihelix: The groove in the posterior surfaces of the antihelix body.

Groove of the superior antihelix crus: The depression in the posterior surface of the superior antihelix crus.

Groove of the inferior antihelix crus: The depression in the posterior surface of the inferior antihelix crus.

Groove of the helix crus: The posterior surface of the helix crus.

Groove of the antitragus: The posterior surface of the antitragus.

Prominence of the scaphoid fossa: The prominence of the posterior surface of the scaphoid fossa.

Prominence of the triangular fossa: The posterior surface of the triangular fossa, i. e., the prominence between the groove of the superior antihelix crus and the groove of the inferior antihelix crus.

Prominence of the superior concha: The prominence of the posterior surface of the superior concha.

Prominence of the inferior concha: The prominence of the posterior surface of the inferior concha.

Ⅱ. Concept and Distributive Regularity of Auricular Points

1. Concept

Auricular points are the sites where the function of the Zang-Fu organs, Channels and Collaterals, tissues and organs, four limbs and all bones reflex themselves on the auricle. They are also the points where we apply various stimuli to treat disease.

2. Distributive regularity

Although there are many auricular points on the small auricle, they are distributed regularly. On the anterior surface, the distribution of auricular points is just like an inverted fetus in the womb, with the head downwards, buttocks and legs upwards, and chest and trunk in the middle. The detailed regularity of distribution is as follows: Points located at the antitragus and ear lobe are related to the head and face, those in the scaphoid fossa to the upper limbs, those at the antihelix to the trunk, those at the superior and inferior antihelix crura to the lower limbs and buttocks, those in the triangular fossa to the organs of the pelvis, those around the helix crus to the digestive tract, those in the superior concha to the organs of the abdominal cavity, those in the inferior concha to the organs of the thoracic cavity, those at the tragus to the nasopharynx, and those in the intertragus notch to the endocrine (Fig. 2—3).

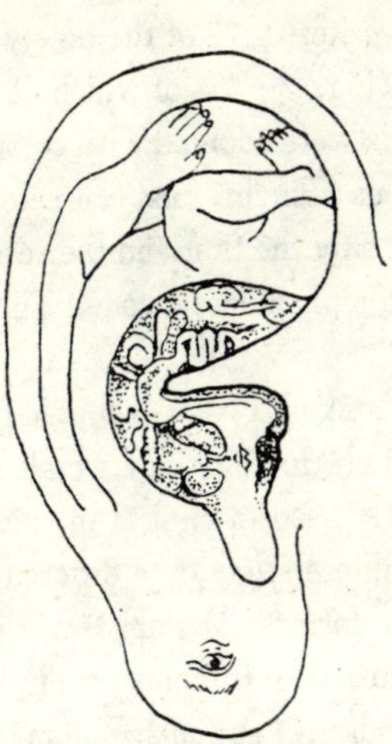

Fig. 2—3 Distributive regularity of auricular points

Ⅲ. Location, Function and indication of Auricular Points

The numbers of auricular points is still controversial, ranging from several decades to several hundred according to statistics. In 1986, All-China Association of Acupuncture and Moxibustion was empowered by the WHO Regional Office for the Western Pacific to lay down a draft The Scheme of International Standardization of Auricular Points. A total of ninety points are adopted in this scheme. In June from 25th to 30th, 1987, WHO Regional Office for the Western Pacific held the Third WHO Regional Working Group Meeting on the Standardization of Acupuncture Nomenclature in Seoul. The main criteria for selection of points were made in the meeting: ① Points which had international and common names in use; ② Points whose therapeutic value well proved; and ③ Points whose location in the auricular area appeared to be generally accepted. According to this criteria, 79 of the ninety points originally presented were adopted (Fig. 2—4), of which 43 points which fulfilled the above three criteria were adopted with complete standardization, i. e. , alphanumeric code, Pinyin, Han characters and English name, and 36 which fulfilled only the first and the second criteria were also adopted but not given alphanumeric code. The remaining 11 points were not accepted.

On the bases of the standard points adopted by All-China Association of Acupuncture and Moxibustion, we also introduce some empirical points frequently used in clinical practice. However, to distinguish them and facilitate study, the different auricular points are marked with different forms: ① Points which fulfilled the above three criteria are marked with combined coding of MA (M indicates micro-system and A indicates auricular points), capitalized first letter of the English name of the actual anatomical area, and alphanumeric coding; ② Points which are adopted by All-China Association of Acupuncture and Moxibustion but not given alphanumeric coding are marked with combined coding of MA and capitalized first letter capitalized first letter of the English name of the actual anatomical area; and ③ Points which frequently used in clinical practice in China but have not adopted by All-China Association of Acupuncture and Moxibustion are marked only with MA.

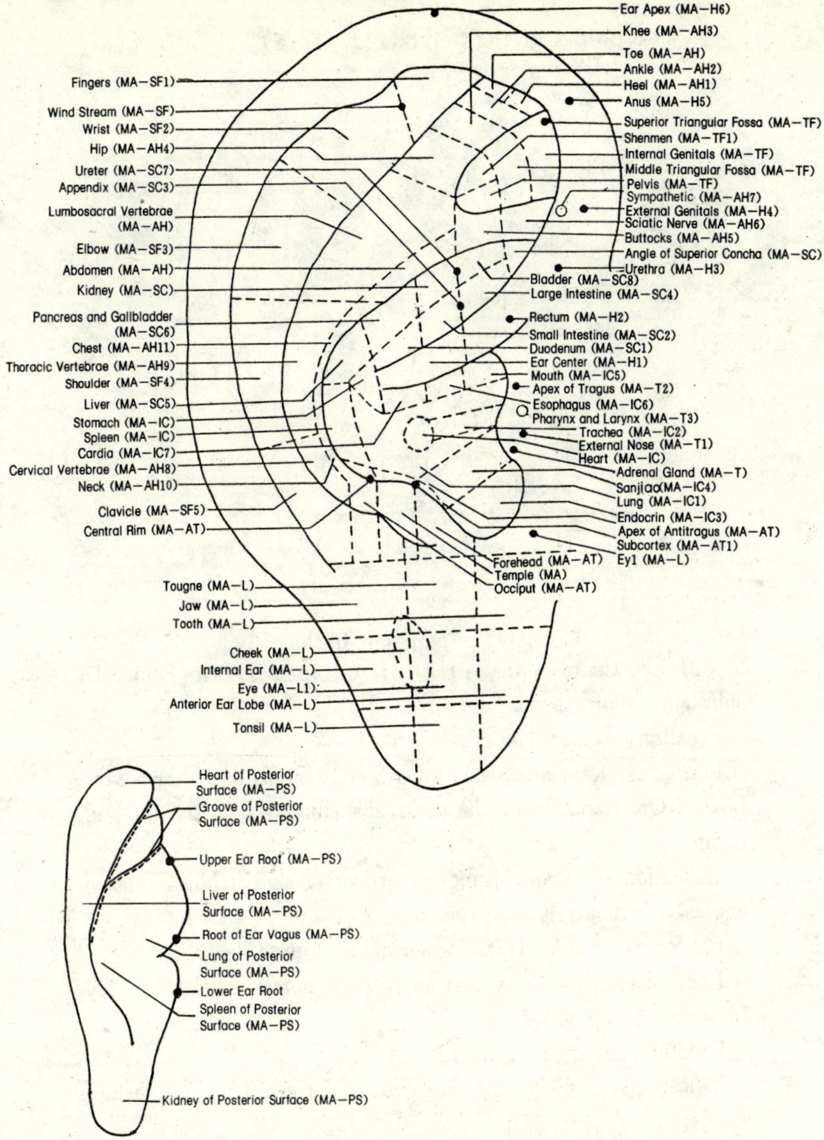

Fig. 2—4 Auricular points adopted by the WHO Regional Office for the Pacific (1987)

1. The points of the helix (Fig. 2—5)

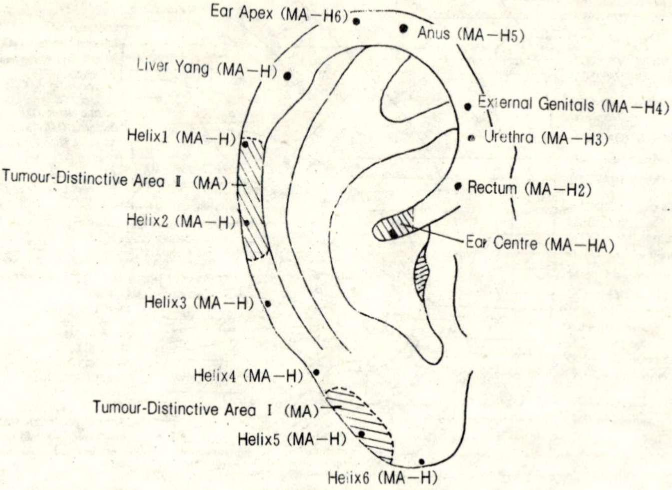

Fig. 2—5 The points of the helix

(1) Ear Center (MA—H1) (former name: Zero Point, Diaphragm, Neurasthenia Point)

Location: At the helix crus.

Functions: Regulating the Stomach and sending down the adverse flow of Qi, tranquilizing the mind, dispelling Wind, and arresting itching.

Indications: Hiccup, jaundice, urticaria, skin itching, infantile enuresis, hemoptysis, and epistaxis.

(2) Rectum (MA—H2) (former name: Lower Rectum)

Location: At the helix near supratragal notch, level with Large Intestine (MA—SC4).

Functions: Regulating the Intestine.

Indications: Constipation, diarrhea, prolapse of anus, and hemorrhoids.

(3) Urethra (MA—H3)

Location: At the helix, superior to Rectum (MA—H2), level

with Bladder (MA—SC8).

Functions: Relieving inflammation and pain and promoting urination.

Indications: Frequent, urgent and painful urination, enuresis, and retention of urine.

(4) External Genitals (MA—H4)

Location: At the helix, superior to Urethra (MA—H3), level with Sympathetic (MA—AH7).

Functions: Clearing away Heat and Dampness, dispelling Wind, and arresting itching.

Indications: Orchitis, epididymitis, pruritus of vulva, swelling and pain of external genitals, and impotence.

(5) Anus (MA—H5)

Locations: At the helix, opposite to the anterior rim of the superior antihelix crus.

Functions: Clearing away Heat and Dampness and relieving inflammation and pain.

Indications: Hemorrhoids, anal fissure, and perianal pruritis.

(6) Ear Apex (MA—H6)

Location: At the top of the helix, opposite to the posterior border of the superior antihelix crus.

Functions: Dispelling Wind and clearing away Heat, relieving inflammation and pain, and calming the Liver to stop convulsion.

Indications: Fever, hypertension, acute conjunctivitis, acute hordeolum, acne, acute tonsillitis, and neurosism

(7) Liver Yang (MA—H)

Location: At the helix tubercle.

Functions: Clearing away Heat and Toxic Materials, calming the Liver and suppressing the hyperactivity of Yang.

Indications: Dizziness, headache, hypertension, and acute conjunctivitis.

(8) Helix 1—6 (MA—H)

Location: Divide the helix area into five equal parts from the lower border of the helix tubercle to the midpoint of the lower border of the ear lobe. The points making the divisions are respectively named

Helix 1, 2, 3, 4, 5 and 6.

Functions: Clearing away Heat and Toxic Materials and relieving swelling and pain.

Indications: Fever, tonsillitis, hypertension, and infection of the upper respiratory tract.

(9) Tumour-Distinctive Area1 (MA)

Location: In the lower part of helix, at the upper two thirds portion of the line connecting the junction, the intersection of the helix and the extension line from Stomach (MA—IC) to the antihelix-antitragus notch, and Helix6 (MA—H).

Functions and indications: A reference point for diagnosis of malignant tumour.

(10) Tumour-Distinctive Area2 (MA)

Location: In the middle part of the helix, at the upper two thirds of the line connecting Helix1 (MA—H) and Helix3 (MA—H).

Functions and indications: A reference point for diagnosis of malignant tumour, especially digestive tumour.

2. The points of the scaphoid fossa (Fig. 2—6)

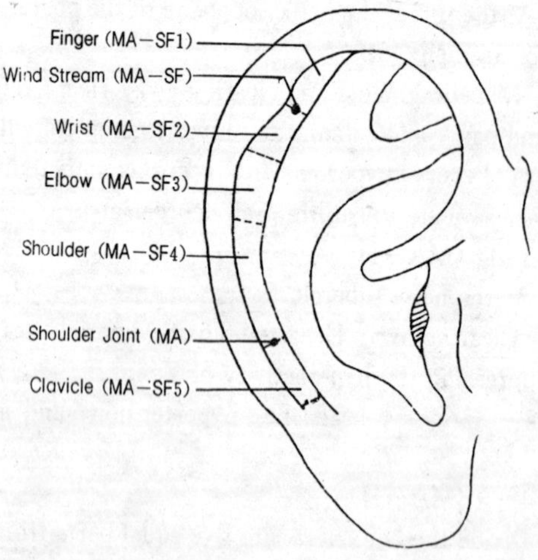

Fig. 2—6 The points of the scaphoid fossa

To facilitate point location, the scaphoid fossa is divided into six equal portions from upward to downward.

(1) Finger (MA—SF1)

Location: The first portion of the scapha.

Functions: Dredging Collaterals and stopping pain.

Indications: Paronychia, and pain and numbness of fingers.

(2) Wrist (MA—SF2)

Location: The second portion of the scapha.

Functions: Dredging Collaterals and relieving pain.

Indications: Pain of the wrist region, such as sprain of the wrist and carpal tunnel syndrome. It is also effective for stomachache and allergic dermatitis.

(3) Elbow (MA—SF3)

Location: The third portion of the scapha.

Functions: Dredging Collaterals and relieving pain.

Indications: External humeral epicondylitis and pain of the wrist region.

(4) Shoulder (MA—SF4)

Location: The area between the fourth and the fifth portion of the scapha.

Functions: Dispelling Wind and Cold, dredging Collaterals, and relieving pain.

Indications: Diseases of the shoulder, such as periarthritis of shoulder joint, subacromial bursitis, and paralysis of the upper limb. It is also effective for cholelithiasis.

(5) Clavicle (MA—SF5)

Location: The sixth portion of the scapha.

Functions: Relaxing tendons and muscles, dredging Collaterals, and relieving pain.

Indications: Periarthritis of the shoulder, and pain of the neck and upper back.

(6) Wind Stream (MA—SF)

Location: In the scapha, at the midpoint between Finger (MA—SF1) and Wrist (MA—SF2), in front of the helix tubercle.

Functions: Dispelling Wind and arresting itching, relieving cough and asthma, and checking allergic reaction.

Indications: Dermatoses such as urticaria, eczema, neurodermatitis and cutaneous pruritus, asthma, and allergic rhinitis.

(7) Shoulder Joint (MA)

Location: In the scaphoid fossa, at the mid-point between Shoulder (MA-SF4) and Clavicle (MA-SF5).

Functions: Dispelling Wind and Dampness, activating Blood, and dredging Collaterals.

Indications: Periarthritis of shoulder and subacromial bursitis.

3. The points of the antihelix (Fig. 2-7)

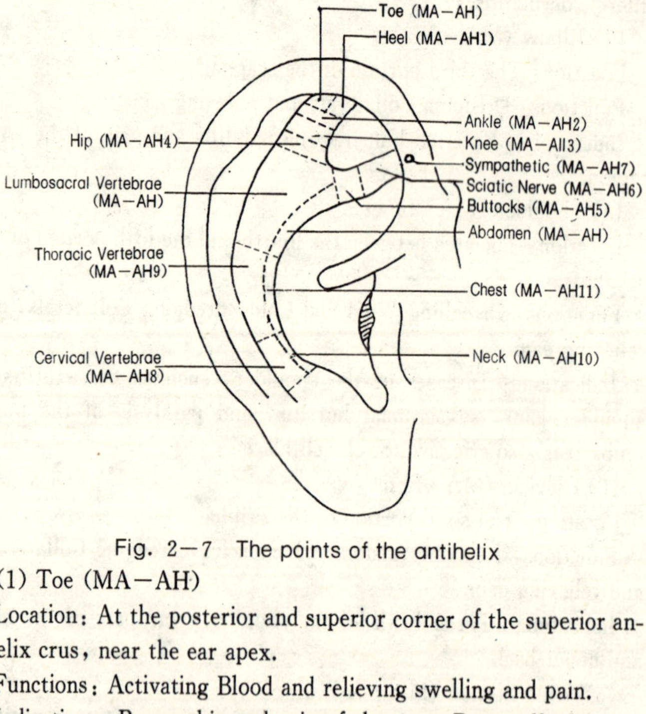

Fig. 2-7 The points of the antihelix

(1) Toe (MA-AH)

Location: At the posterior and superior corner of the superior antihelix crus, near the ear apex.

Functions: Activating Blood and relieving swelling and pain.

Indications: Paronychia and pain of the toes, Raynaud's disease, and erythromelalgia.

(2) Heel (MA-AH1)

Location: At the anterior and superior corner of the superior antihelix crus, near the upper end of the triangular fossa.

Functions: Activating Blood and relieving swelling and pain.

Indications: Heel pain.

(3) Ankle (MA—AH2)

Location: Midway between Heel (MA—AH1) and Knee (MA—AH3).

Functions: Activating Blood and relieving pain.

Indications: Sprain and contusion of the ankle joint.

(4) Knee (MA—AH3)

Location: At the middle one-third portion of the superior antihelix crus.

Functions: Dispelling Wind and Dampness, activating Blood, dredging Collaterals, and relieving pain.

Indications: Swelling and pain of knee joint and rheumatic arthritis.

(5) Hip (MA—AH4)

Location: At the lower one-third portion of the superior antihelix crus

Functions: Activating Blood and relieving pain.

Indications: Pain of the hip joint and sciatica.

(6) Sympathetic (MA—AH7)

Location: At the antihelix, on the junction of the terminal point of the inferior antihelix crus and helix.

Functions: Regulating the function of the sympathetic nerve and parasympathetic nerve, relaxing spasm of smooth muscle and relieving pain.

Indications: Gastrointestinal spasm, angina pectoris, biliary colic, calculi of ureter, dysfunction of the autonomous nervous system, acrotism, and asthma.

(7) Sciatic Nerve (MA—AH6)

Location: At the anterior two-thirds portions of the inferior antihelix crus.

Functions: Activating Blood and dredging Collaterals, removing Blood stasis, and relieving pain.

Indications: Sciatica and paralysis of the lower limb.

(8) Buttocks (MA—AH5)

Location: At the lower one-third portion of the inferior antihelix crus.

Functions: Activating Blood and relieving pain.

Indications: Sciatica and fasciitis of the gluteal region.

(9) Lumbosacral Vertebrae (MA—AH)

Location: A curved line from the antihelix-antitragal notch to the bifurcation of the superior and inferior antihelix crura is divided into five equal segments. Lumbosacral Vertebrae (MA—AH) is located in the upper two fifths of the antihelix.

Functions: Strengthening the loins and replenishing the Kidney, dredging Channels and Collaterals, and relieving pain.

Indications: Pain in the lumbosacral area.

(10) Thoracic Vertebrae (MA—AH9)

Location: In the middle two fifths of the antihelix.

Functions: Dredging Channels and Collaterals and relieving pain.

Indications: Pain in the chest and hypochondria, mastitis, insufficient lactation, ankylosing spondylitis, and premenstrual mammary distention and pain.

(11) Cervical Vertebrae (MA—AH8)

Location: The lower one fifth portion of the antihelix.

Functions: Relaxing tendons and muscles and activating Blood, strengthening bones, dredging Channels and Collaterals, and relieving pain. Indications: Stiffneck and cervical spondylopathy.

(12) Abdomen (MA—AH)

Location: At the upper part of the antihelix, at the anterior aspect of Lumbosacral Vertebrae (MA—AH), near the rim of scapha.

Functions: Regulating gastrointestinal function, dredging Collaterals, and relieving pain.

Indications: Abdominal pain and distention, diarrhea, and acute sprain.

(13) Chest (MA—AH11)

Location: At the middle part of the antihelix, at the anterior aspect of Thoracic Vertebrae (MA—AH9), near the rim of scapha.

Functions: Regulating the flow of Qi and alleviating depression, and relieving inflammation and pain.

Indications: Fullness of the chest, intercostal neuralgia, mastitis, oligogalactia, and hypochondriac pain.

(14) Neck (MA-AH10)

Location: At the lower part of the antihelix, at the anterior aspect of Cervical Vertebrae (MA-AH8), near the rim of scapha.

Functions: Dredging Channels and Collaterals, and relieving inflammation and pain.

Indications: Stiffneck, swelling and pain of the neck, and thyroid enlargement.

4. The points of the triangular fossa (Fig. 2-8)

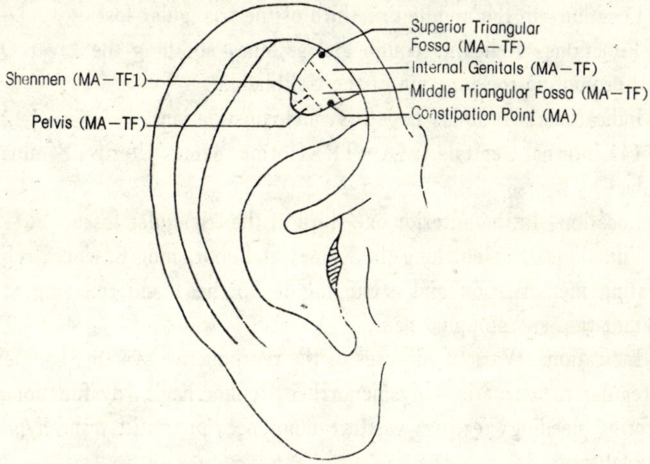

Fig. 2-8 The points of the triangular fossa

(1) Shenmen (MA-TF1)

Location: In the triangular fossa, at the superior aspect of the bifurcating point between the superior and the inferior antihelix crura.

Functions: Calming the Heart and tranquilizing the mind, relieving spasm and pain, alleviating inflammation and itching, and subduing fever.

Indications: Insomnia and dream-disturbed sleep; pain syndromes such as headache, toothache, angina pectoris and neuralgia; various kinds of fever and withdrawal syndromes; and allergic diseases, such as urticaria, pruritis and asthma.

(2) Pelvis (MA—TF)

Location: In the triangular fossa, slightly inferior to the medial side of the bifurcating point between the superior and the inferior antihelix crura.

Functions: Relieving inflammation and pain and regulating menstruation.

Indications: Pelvic inflammation, annexitis, and irregular menstruation.

(3) Middle Triangular Fossa (MA—TF) (former name: Asthma Point and Hepatitis Point)

Location: In the middle one-third of the triangular fossa.

Functions: Relieving cough and asthma, soothing the Liver Qi and promoting the function of the Gallbladder.

Indications: Asthma, hepatitis, and constipation.

(4) Internal Genitals (MA—TF) (former name: Uterus, Seminal Palace)

Location: In the anterior one-third of the triangular fossa.

Functions: Replenishing the Kidney and nourishing Essence, regulating menstruation and astringing leukorrhea, and relieving inflammation and stopping pain.

Indications: Various diseases of the reproductive system, such as irregular menstruation, dysmenorrhea, leukorrhagia, dysfunctional uterine bleeding, testitis, vasitis, impotence, prostatitis, and hyposexuality.

(5) Superior Triangular Fossa (MA—TF) (former name: Lowering Blood Pressure Point)

Location: Anterior and superior of the triangular fossa.

Functions: Lowering blood pressure.

Indications: Hypertension.

(6) Constipation Point (MA)

Location: In the triangular fossa, near the lower border of the fossa, superior to Sciatica (MA—AH6) or the middle portion of the inferior antihelix crus.

Functions: Regulating the Intestine to relax bowels.

Indications: Constipation.

5. The points of the tragus (Fig. 2—9)

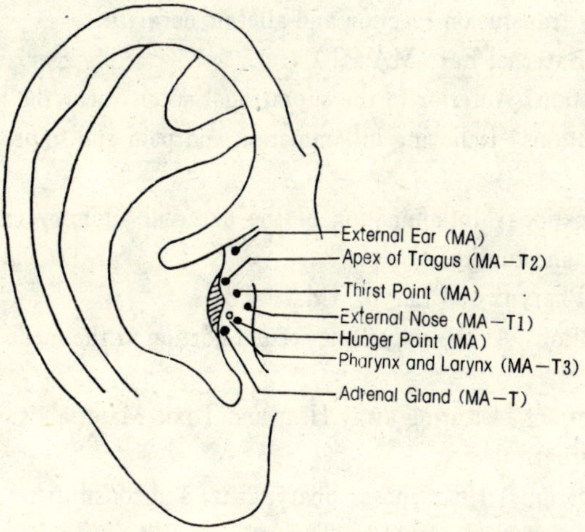

Fig. 2—9 The points of the tragus

(1) External Nose (MA—T1)

Location: At the anterior to the center of the lateral aspect of the tragus.

Functions: Relieving inflammation and pain, and clearing the nasal passage.

Indications: Nasal vestibulitis, rhinitis, and rosacea.

(2) Apex of Tragus (MA—T2)

Location: At the tip of the upper protuberance, on the border of the tragus.

Functions: Subduing fever and relieving pain.

Indications: Fever and toothache.

(3) Adrenal Gland (MA—T)

Location: At the tip of the lower protuberance on the border of the tragus.

Functions: Relieving inflammation and pain, regulating the secretion of the adrenaline, relieving cough and asthma, clearing away Heat and Dampness, alleviating spasm and pain, expelling Wind, and arresting itching.

Indications: Hypotension, rheumatic arthritis, parotitis, tertian malaria, streptomycin toxic dizziness, asthma, and allergic diseases such as transfusion reaction and allergic dermatitis.

(4) External Ear (MA—T)

Location: Anterior to the supratragal notch, near the helix.

Functions: Relieving inflammation and pain and improving hearing.

Indications: Inflammation of the external auditory canal, otitis media, and tinnitus.

(5) Pharynx and Larynx (MA—T3)

Location: At the upper one second portion of the medial aspect of tragus.

Functions: Clearing away Heat and Toxic Materials and relieving sore throat.

Indications: Hoarseness, pharyngitis, and tonsillitis.

(6) Internal Nose (MA—T)

Location: At the lower one second portion of the medial aspect of tragus.

Functions: Clearing away Heat and Toxic Materials and clearing the nasal passage.

Indications: Rhinitis, paranasal sinusitis, epistaxis, and nasal obstruction due to cold.

(7) Thirst Point (MA)

Location: At the midway between External Nose (MA—T1) and Apex of Tragus (MA—T2).

Functions: Nourishing Yin and promoting the production of body fluid to relieve thirst.

Indications: Diabetes mellitus, diabetes insipidus, and neurogenic polydipsia.

(8) Hunger Point (MA)

Location: At the midway between External Nose (MA—T1) and

Adrenal Gland (MA—T).

Functions: Regulating endocrine and reducing appetite.

Indications: Obesity and hyperthyroidism.

6. The points of the antitragus (Fig. 2—10)

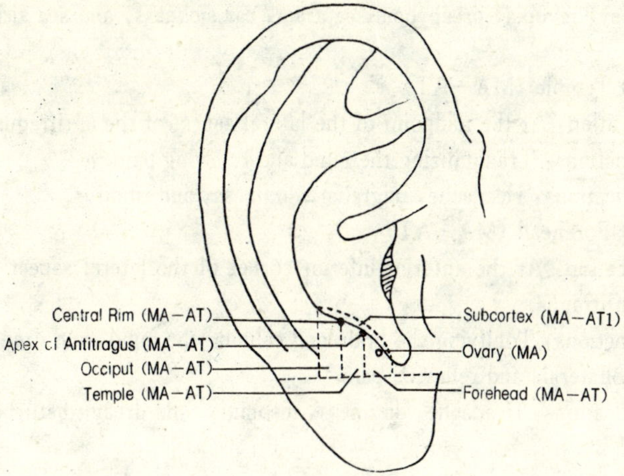

Fig. 2—10 The points of the antitragus

(1) Apex of Antitragus (MA—AT)

Location: At the tip of the antitragus.

Functions: Relieving cough and asthma, subduing inflammation, ceasing pain, dispelling Wind, and arresting itching.

Indications: Asthma, mumps, cutaneous pruritus, testitis, and epididymitis.

(2) Central Rim (MA—AT) (former name: brain point)

Location: At the midpoint between the antitragal apex and antihelix- antitragal notch.

Functions: Nourishing brain and tranquilizing the mind.

Indications: Intellectual disturbance, enuresis, diabetes insipidus, auditory vertigo, irregular menstruation, dysfunctional uterine bleeding, and shock.

(3) Occiput (MA—AT)

Location: At the posterior-superior corner of the lateral aspect of the antitragus.

Functions: Tranquilizing the mind and calming the Heart, checking Wind and relieving spasm, and nourishing the Liver and improving vision.

Indications: Dizziness, vertigo, headache, insomnia, asthma, epilepsy, myopia, presbyopia, cataract, car sickness, and sea sickness.

(4) Temple (MA−AT)

Location: At the midpoint of the lateral aspect of the antitragus.

Functions: Tranquilizing the mind and relieving pain.

Indications: Headache, migraine, dizziness, and tinnitus.

(5) Forehead (MA−AT)

Location: At the anterior-inferior corner of the lateral aspect of the antitragus.

Functions: Tonifying the brain and calming the mind, and dredging Collaterals and relieving pain.

Indications: Headache, dizziness, insomnia, and dream-disturbed sleep.

(6) Subcortex (MA−AT1)

Location: On the medial aspect of the antitragus.

Functions: Tonifying the brain, calming the mind, and relieving inflammation and pain. The point has the efficacy of regulating the excito- inhibitory function of the cerebral cortex.

Indications: Pain syndromes, tertian malaria, neurosism, dream-disturbed sleep, pseudomyopia, inflammation and dysfunction of the vegetative nerve. Subcortex (MA−AT1) is one of the most common auricular points used for auricular acupuncture anesthesia.

(7) Ovary (MA)

Location: In the interior aspect of antitragus, the medial side of the line from the apex to the bottom of antitragus, near Endocrine (MA−IC3).

Functions: Regulating menstruation, enriching Blood, tonifying the Kidney, and replenishing Essence.

Indications: Irregular menstruation and hypogonadia.

7. The points of the inferior concha (Fig. 2—11)

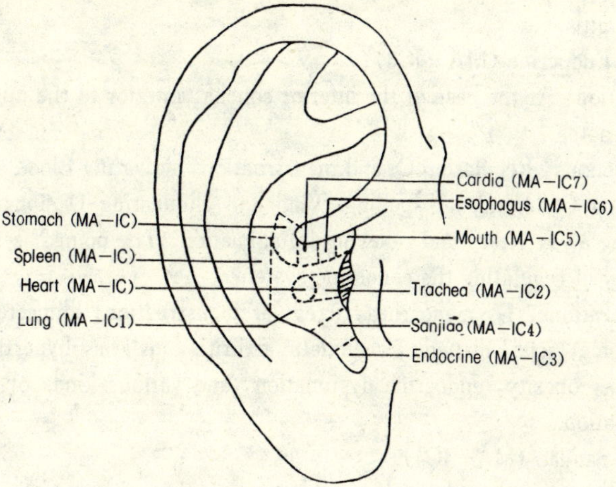

Fig. 2—11 The points of the inferior concha

(1) Heart (MA—IC)

Location: In the central depression of the inferior concha.

Functions: Calming the Heart and tranquilizing the mind.

Indications: Tachycardia, arrhythmia, angina pectoris, acrotism, neurasthenia, insomnia, schizophrenia, stomatitis, and ulceration of the mouth and tongue.

(2) Lung (MA—IC1)

Location: Around the central depression or Heart (MA—IC) of the inferior concha.

Functions: Relieving cough and asthma, dispelling Wind, and arresting itching.

Indications: Cough, asthma, chest stuffiness, hoarseness, laryngitis, acne, flat wart, urticaria, skin pruritus, constipation, withdrawal syndrome, and rhinitis.

(3) Trachea (MA—IC2)

Location: Between the orifice of the external auditory meatus and Heart (MA—IC).

Functions: Relieving cough and asthma, clearing away Heat, and dissolving phlegm.

Indications: Cough, asthma, bronchitis, and acute or chronic pharyngitis.

(4) Endocrine (MA—IC3)

location: At the base of the inferior concha, interior to the intertragal notch.

Functions: Regulating Qi and menstruation, activating Blood and dredging Collaterals, dispelling Wind and eliminating Dampness, clearing away Heat, and relieving inflammation. The point has the efficacy of regulating the endocrine system.

Indications: Dysmenorrhea, irregular menstruation, climacteric syndrome, acne, diabetes, rheumatic arthritis, malaria, hyperthyroidism, obesity, endocrine dysfunction, and various kinds of inflammation.

(5) Sanjiao (MA—IC4)

Location: At the base of the inferior concha, superior to Endocrine (MA—IC3).

Functions: Regulating the Intestine and clearing the Water Passage.

Indications: Constipation, abdominal distention, edema, diabetes, and pain of the lateral aspect of the upper limb.

(6) Spleen (MA—IC)

Location: At the posterior and superior aspect of the inferior concha.

Functions: Strengthening the Spleen and the Stomach, invigorating Qi in the Middle Jiao, and regulating menstruation.

Indications: Abdominal distention, diarrhea, anorexia, dysfunctional uterine bleeding, leukorrhagia, proctoptosis, and auditory vertigo.

(7) Stomach (MA—IC)

Location: Around the area where the helix terminates.

Functions: Regulating the Stomach to stop vomiting and promoting the flow of Qi to relieve pain.

Indications: Gastrospasm, gastritis. gastric ulcer, indigestion, dysfunction of gastrointestinal tract, insomnia, and toothache. It is also effective for epilepsy, schizophrenia and hysteria.

(8) Cardia (MA-IC7)

Location: At the lateral one-third portion of the inferior aspect of the helix crus.

Functions: Regulating the Stomach to arrest vomiting.

Indications: Cardiospasm and nervous vomiting.

(9) Esophagus (MA-IC6)

Location: At the middle two-thirds portion of the inferior aspect of the helix crus.

Functions: Regulating the flow of Qi to ease chest oppression and relieve inflammation and spasm.

Indications: Esophagitis, esophageal spasm, and dyspnea.

(10) Mouth (MA-IC5)

Location: At the anterior one-third portion of the inferior aspect of the helix crus.

Functions: Dredging Channels and Collaterals, clearing away Heat and Toxic Materials, relieving inflammation and pain and regulating one's taste.

Indications: Facial paralysis, stomatitis, cholecystitis, cholelithiasis, and withdrawal syndrome.

8. The points of the superior concha (Fig. 2-12)

(1) Duodenum (MA-SC1)

Location: In the superior concha, posterior and superior to the helix crus.

Functions: Relieving spasm and stopping pain.

Indications: Duodenal ulcer, pylorospasm, cholecystitis, and cholelithiasis.

(2) Small Intestine (MA-SC2)

Location: In the superior concha, at the superior and middle aspect of the helix crus.

Functions: Regulating the Intestine, promoting digestion, calming the Heart, and tranquilizing the mind.

Indications: Indigestion, abdominal pain or distention, diarrhea, and gastrointestinal dysfunction. It is also effective for tachycardia, arrhythmia and oligogalactia.

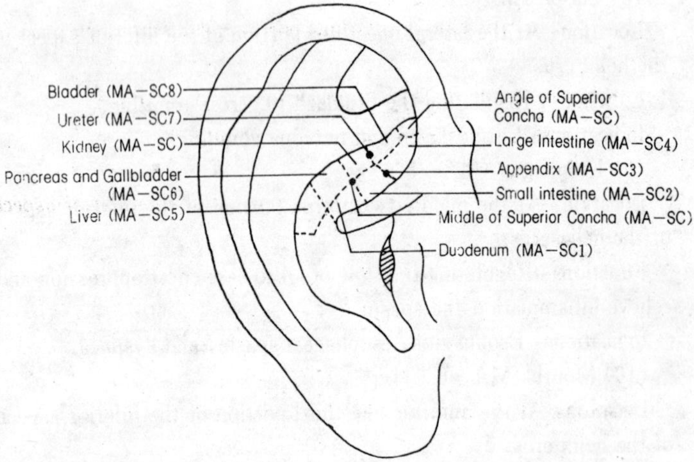

Fig. 2-12 The points of the superior concha

(3) Large Intestine (MA-SC4)

Location: In the superior concha, at the medial 1/3 section of the superior aspect of the helix crus.

Functions: Regulating the Intestine to relieve constipation or diarrhea.

Indications: Diarrhea, constipation, and dysentery. It is also effective for cough, acne, and nasopharyngeal disease.

(4) Appendix (MA-SC3)

Location: In the superior concha, between Small Intestine (MA-SC2) and Large Intestine (MA-SC4).

Functions: Relieving inflammation and ceasing pain.

Indications: Simple appendicitis and diarrhea.

(5) Liver (MA-SC5)

Location: In the superior concha, at the lateral inferior portion of the superior concha.

Functions: Easing the depressed Liver and promoting the function of the Gallbladder, enriching Blood to improve vision, and regulating Qi to relieve depression.

Indications: Hypochondriac pain, dizziness, premenstrual syndrome, climacteric syndrome, hypertension, pseudomyopia, simple glaucoma, cholecystitis, cholelithiasis, acute conjunctivitis, and neurosism.

(6) Pancreas and Gallbladder (MA−SC6)

Location: In the superior concha, between Liver (MA−SC5) and Kidney (MA−SC).

Functions: Easing the depressed Liver and promoting the function of the Gallbladder, clearing away Heat and removing Toxic Materials, and dredging Collaterals and relieving pain.

Indications: Cholecystitis, cholelithiasis, biliary ascariasis, migraine, herpes zoster, otitis media, tinnitus, poor hearing, acute pancreasitis, and diabetes mellitus.

(7) Kidney (MA−SC)

Location: In the superior concha, inferior to the bifurcating point between superior antihelix crus and inferior antihelix crus.

Functions: Tonifying the Kidney, enriching Essence, clearing and regulating Water Passage, and improving vision and hearing.

Indications: Lumbago, tinnitus, neurosism, pyelonephritis, asthma, enuresis, irregular menstruation, spermatorrhea, premature ejaculation, and diarrhea resulting from Kidney deficiency.

(8) Ureter (MA−SC7)

Location: In the superior concha between Kidney (MA−SC) and Bladder (MA−SC8).

Functions: Clearing away Heat-Dampness from the Lower Jiao, relieving spasm, and stopping pain.

Indications: Colic pain due to ureter calculi, and urinary tract infection.

(9) Bladder (MA−SC8)

Location: In the superior concha, between Kidney (MA−SC) and Angle of Superior Concha (MA−SC).

Functions: Clearing away Heat-Dampness from the Lower Jiao and dredging Channels and Collaterals.

Indications: Cystitis, enuresis, retention of urine, lower back pain, sciatica, occipital pain, and urinary calculi.

(10) Angle of Superior Concha (MA−SC)

Location: At the medial superior angle of the superior concha.

Functions: Clearing away Heat, eliminating Dampness, replenishing the Kidney, and enriching Essence.

Indications: Prostatitis, prostatic hyperplasia, urethritis, and sexual disorder.

(11) Middle of Superior Concha (MA—SC)

Location: In the center of the superior concha.

Functions: Clearing away Heat, relieving pain, regulating the Middle Jiao, and replenishing the Spleen.

Indications: Abdominal pain and distention, biliary ascariasis, and parotitis.

9. The points of the ear lobe (Fig. 2—13)

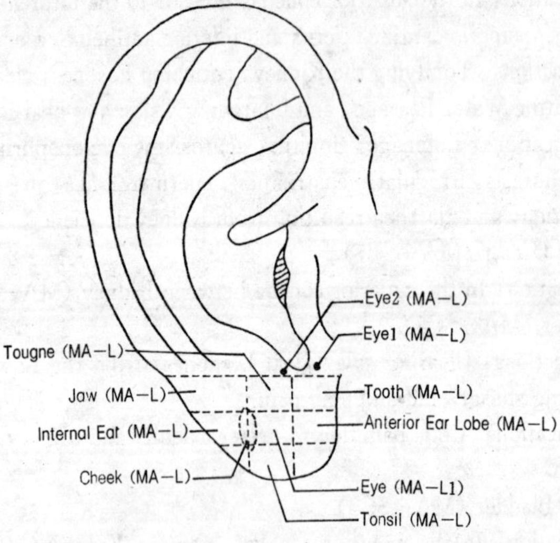

Fig. 2—13 The points of the ear lobe

To facilitate the location of points, the ear lobe is divided into nine parts. Draw three proportional and horizontal lines from the lower border of the cartilage of the intertragal notch to the inferior rim of the ear lob, draw another two vertical and proportional lines from the second horizontal line. The ear lobe is divided into nine areas from anterior to posterior and from upward to downward.

(1) Eye1 (MA−L)

Location: On the anterior and inferior sides of the intertragal notch.

Functions: Enriching Essence to improve eyesight.

Indications: Pseudomyopia.

(2) Eye2 (MA−L)

Location: On the posterior and inferior aspect of the intertragal notch.

Functions: Enriching Essence to improve eyesight

Indications: Pseudomyopia.

(3) Tooth (MA−L)

Location: In the first area.

Functions: Relieving inflammation, stopping pain, invigorating Qi, and enriching Blood.

Indications: Toothache, periodontitis, and hypotension.

(4) Tongue (MA−L)

Location: In the second area.

Functions: Relieving inflammation and stopping pain.

Indications: Glossitis and stomatitis.

(5) Jaw (MA−L)

Location: In the third area.

Functions: Relieving inflammation, stopping pain, and dredging Channels and Collaterals.

Indications: Toothache and dysfunction of the tempomandibular joint.

(6) Anterior Ear Lobe (MA−L)

Location: In the fourth area.

Functions: Calming the Heart, tranquilizing the mind, relieving inflammation, and stopping pain.

Indications: Neurasthenia and toothache.

(7) Eye (MA−L1)

Location: In the fifth area.

Functions: Clearing away Heat, removing Toxic Materials, nourishing the Liver, and improving vision.

Indications: Acute conjunctivitis, electric ophthalmia, hordeolum, and pseudomyopia.

(8) Internal Ear (MA—L)

Location: In the sixth area.

Functions: Replenishing the Liver and the Kidney, enriching Blood, and improving hearing.

Indications: Internal auditory vertigo, tinnitus, and poor hearing.

(9) Tonsil (MA—L)

Location: In the eighth area.

Functions: Clearing away Heat and Toxic Materials and relieving sore throat.

Indications: Tonsillitis and pharyngitis.

(10) Cheek (MA—L)

Location: Around the juncture between the fifth area and the sixth area.

Functions: Dispelling Wind, dredging Collaterals, relieving inflammation, and stopping pain.

Indications: Facial paralysis, trigeminal neuralgia, acne, and flat wart.

10. The points of the posterior auricular surface (Fig. 2—14)

(1) Upper Ear Root (MA—PS)

Location: At the upper most rim of the root of ear.

Functions: Relieving pain and asthma and arresting bleeding.

Indications: headache, asthma, epistaxis, and paralysis.

(2) Root of Ear Vagus (MA—PS)

Location: Corresponding to the helix crus, at the root of the ear or the junction between the ear back and mastoid process.

Functions: Clearing away Heat and Dampness and relieving spasm and pain.

Indications: Cholecystitis, cholelithiasis, biliary ascariasis, tachycardia, abdominal pain, diarrhea, and nasal obstruction.

(3) Lower Ear Root (MA—PS)

Location: At the lower most rim of the root of ear.

Functions: Invigorating Qi, regulating Blood, and tranquilizing the mind.

Indications: Hypotension.

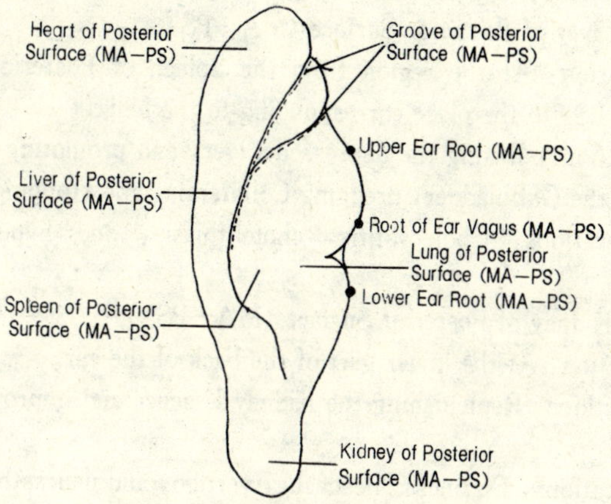

Fig. 2—14 The points of the posterior auricular surface

(4) Groove of Posterior Surface (MA—PS)

Location: In a "Y" form depression on the back of the ear, which is surrounded by and corresponding to the antihelix, superior antihelix crus and inferior antihelix crus.

Functions: Calming the Liver, sending down the adverse flow of the Liver Qi, dispelling Wind, and relieving itching.

Indications: Hypertension and cutaneous pruritus.

(5) Heart of Posterior Surface (MA—PS)

Location: At the upper part of the back of the ear

Functions: Calming the Heart and tranquilizing the mind.

Indications: Palpitation, insomnia, and dream-disturbed sleep.

(6) Lung of Posterior Surface (MA—PS)

Location: At the region from Spleen of Posterior Surface (MA—PS) to the root of the ear.

Functions: Relieving cough and asthma, dispelling Wind, and arresting itching.

Indications: Cough, asthma, and cutaneous pruritis.

(7) Spleen of Posterior Surface (MA—PS)

Location: At the back region where the helix crus terminates.

Functions: Replenishing the Spleen and the Stomach.

Indications: Stomachache, indigestion, and anorexia.

(8) Liver of Posterior Surface (MA—PS)

Location: At the region from the Spleen of Posterior Surface (MA—PS) to the place corresponding to the helix.

Functions: Easing the depressed Liver, and promoting the function of the Gallbladder, dredging Collaterals, and stopping pain.

Indications: Cholecystitis, cholelithiasis, and hypochondriac pain.

(9) Kidney of Posterior Surface (MA—PS)

Location: At the lower part of the back of the ear.

Functions: Replenishing the Kidney Essence and improving hearing.

Indications: Dizziness, headache, vertigo, and neurasthenia.

Auricular Diagnosis

TCM holds that the activities of the internal organs must reflect themselves on the outside of the body. As early as the *Nei Jing* (Internal Classic) times, the ear was used to diagnose diseases. The chapter *Wei Qi Shi Chang Pian* (Dysfunction of the Defensive Qi) of *Ling Shu* (Miraculous Pivot) states that withered ear suggests a disease of the bone. However, records in the ancient works are not systematic. Only in recent several decades has the knowledge of auricular diagnosis developed rapidly and exibited its unique charms.

Ⅰ. Diagnostic Methods

1. Inspection

A diagnostic method achieved by observing alterations of color, shape, skin rash, furfures, angioplerosis, etc. in the auricle.

When observing the auricle, the following precautions should be paid:

(1) Excessive stimulation to the auricle before observation should be avoided, wash and sterilization as well. If there is too much dirt

on the ear which affects the inspection, ask the patient to clean it with clear water one or two days before examination.

(2) Natural light is adopted as much as possible when observing. When observing some depressions on the auricle such as triangular fossa and superior concha, support the ear with the middle finger from the back of the ear and separate the helix crus or antihelix crus with a detective bar in order to fully expose the observed area.

(3) Holding the auricle gently with the index finger and thumb, the medical worker uses level eye-sight when observing and searching for positive matters according to the anatomical order of the auricle (i. e., from inner to lateral and from upper to lower).

(4) When a susceptible positive matter is found, to ascertain its nature and significance, one should observe the corresponding area carefully with the index finger or middle finger supporting the auricle from the posterior surface of the auricle and the thumb touching the vicinity of the positive matter to stretch the auricle gently upwards, downwards and laterally.

2. Pressing

A method performed by pressing auricular points with a probe to detect the sensitive points and therefore assisting to establish a diagnosis. When performing this examination, one should pay attention to the detecting order and pressing force. The detecting order is usually from upper to lower, and from inner to lateral or from lateral to inner to avoid omitting some points. The pressing force should be even and proper to find out the most pain-sensitive point. Since pain is a kind of subjective feeling from patients, the pressing force should be different with different persons, generally smaller to the sensitive ones and bigger to the insensitive ones.

3. Palpation

Holding the ear with the thumb and index finger: the index finger on the posterior side and the thumb on the detected auricular point, the doctor palpates the selected point with these two fingers laying strength oppositely and cooperatively. Palpation is chosen mainly for the purpose of observing the morphologic alteration of the subcutaneous tissues, e.g., prominence, depression, node, etc.

4. Pressing mark method

When morphological changes are present in auricular points, traces will be left following pressing the points with probe. Observing the different marks such as depth of the mark and change of color is helpful to establishing a diagnosis.

5. Measurement of electric property

There are various electric detectors of auricular points that can be used to measure the electrical resistance, voltage, current and electric capacity, etc. Generally speaking, the auricular points associated with the disease have lower electrical resistance and higher current, compared with unconcerned points. Before testing, pressing and kneading the auricle or washing it with water or alcohol should be avoided in case causing local congestion leading to false reactants. If too much dirt on the ear, clean it with soap water or clear water, dry it with cotton ball, and then give the test ten minutes later.

6. Dyeing

Based on the theory of biological histochemical stain, auricular points associated a disease can be dyed with colorful organic compounds while those unconcerned can not be dyed. This method is suitable for diagnosis of chronic diseases.

There are lots of prescriptions of dye liquid available at present. Here we recommend a prescription formulated by Yunnan Institute of Auricular Acupuncture for reference.

Ingredients:

Eriochrome black T: 0.2g

Gentian violet: 1.0g

Aniline: 2.0g

99% alcohol: 90 ml

Dyeing process:

(1) Cleaning: First the sebaceous substance on the auricular skin

is removed with 5% sedium bicarbonate. Then the dirt is cleaned by oxidization with 0. 25% potassium permanganate, followed by reduction with 5% oxalic acid solution. Finally the auricle is washed with distilled water and dried softly with cotton ball.

(2) Dyeing: Paint the anterior auricular surface three times within 30 seconds with cotton ball which fully absorbs dyeing liquid. Then clean the liquid with 95% alcohol cotton ball two times till most of the surface restores to original color. Observe auricular points after the auricle is dried with cotton ball.

Ⅱ. Pathological Reactions of Auricular Points

Diseases in human body usually show abnormal pathological reactions on the corresponding area of the auricle, some of which can be observed by naked eyes while some measured by advice. According to clinical observation, commonly-seen pathological reactions are as follows: tenderness, desquamation, red spot, small blister, congestion, local edema, bleeding point, scar, prominence, depression, fold, etc. Different pathological reactions indicate different pathological changes of the disease.

1. Manifestations and significance

(1) Color changes: It refers to skin color at the locus of the auricular points differing from the surrounding normal skin. The changed color may be spot-shaped or patch-shaped pale, dark red, grey, or dark brown, etc. Color change is frequently encountered in inflammatory diseases, e.g., gastritis, enteritis, appendicitis, pneumonia, nephritis, cystitis, arthritis, etc. In addition, it is also seen in hypertension and some gynecological diseases. As a rule, spot-shaped or patch-shaped redness and red papula with lustrous greasy surface suggest an acute inflammatory disease while those with dull color indicate a chronic inflammatory disease.

(2) Shape changes: It refers to morphological changes of the area of auricular points. Main changes of shape include local prominence, depression and fold with a shape of node, cycle, spot or strip. Shape changes indicate organic diseases, e.g., hepatosplenomegaly, hepatitis, cirrhosis, tuberculosis, tumor and congenital heart disease.

(3) Papule: It refers to spot-shaped prominence of the auricular point area. The papula may be reddish, whitish or blister-like and are often seen in organic or inflammatory diseases, e.g., chronic nephritis, cystitis, urinary infection and chronic bronchitis. Generally, reddish papule with lustrous greasy surface indicate an acute inflammatory change while whitish papule with dull color or desquamation on surface indicate a chronic inflammatory change.

(4) Desquamation: It refers to furfuraceous desquamation presenting in the area of auricular points, which is somewhat difficult to be removed. Desquamation is often seen in various dermatoses, gynecological diseases and some chronic inflammatory diseases, e.g., cutaneous pruritis, neurodermatitis, etc. It can also be seen in patients suffering from insomnia, constipation or climacteric syndrome.

(5) Angioplerosis: It refers to excessive angioplerosis or angiectasis in the locus of auricular points. Angioplerosis is most commonly seen in diseases of the circulatory system and acute inflammation, e.g., hypertension, coronary arteriosclerotic cardiopathy, myocardiac infarction, laryngopharyngitis, tonsillitis and mastitis.

(6) Tenderness: It refers to an obvious pain reaction upon pressure in the area of auricular points. According to severity of pain, tender spot can be classified into four degrees:

Degree Ⅰ: Slight pain.

Degree Ⅱ: Moderate pain. The patient knits his brows when points are pressed.

Degree Ⅲ: Remarkable pain. The patient knits his brows and twists his mouth when points are pressed.

Degree Ⅳ: Severe pain. The patient screams, refuses to be pressed and presents escaping behavior due to intolerable pain. Tenderness is the most common pathological reaction, being seen in all kinds of diseases. It can not only reflect whether or not there is a disease in the body but also suggest the severity and development of the disease.

(7) Change of electric property: It refers to changes of the electric resistance, electric capacity, voltage, or current in the area of auricular points. On normal condition, when a person is ill, electric resistance will decrease while electric capacity increase in the corresponding auricular points. These changes of electric properties can be measured by devices. It is reported that normally the electric resistance is between 1—4 MΩ, electric capacity 0. 001—0. 01 μF, electric current 0. 5211—3. 904 μA, and electric voltage 0. 2146—66. 69 mV. However, at the sensitive auricular points, the electric resistance is between 50—300 KΩ, electric capacity 0. 05—1. 0 μF, electric current 1. 999—36. 08 μA, and electric voltage 10. 39—450. 6 mV.

2. Precautions

When gathering clinical information of the auricular points, more attention should be paid to the followings to distinguish the true reaction from the pseudo one.

(1) Avoiding washing the ear before observation. If there is too much dirt which affects observation, clean the auricle in one direction with dry cotton ball.

(2) Applying plentiful light when observing. Use natural light as far as possible.

(3) Ascertaining the true reaction. In healthy persons, there may be pigmentation, whitish node, small pustule, and scar of injury or frostbite in the auricle without diagnostic significance. A simple method for differentiating a true positive reaction from a pseudo one is to press it. The one with obvious pain upon pressure is the true pathological reaction while the one without pain is in most cases a false reaction.

(4) Paying attention to the differentiation of the pathological tenderness and the physiological one. Physically, pain reaction exists in

all auricular points and it may be rather obvious in some sensitive auricular points, such as Shenmen (MA—TF1) and Sympathetic (MA—AH7). However, the pain reaction is much more severe in pathological condition. Therefore, the key to distinguish them is to have a comparison between different points, and before and after a disease.

Ⅲ. Applications of Auricular Diagnosis

1. Respiratory diseases

Acute bronchitis: Spot-like redness or red papula appear in Trachea (MA—IC2) and Bronchus (MA).

Chronic bronchitis: In the area of Trachea (MA — IC2) or Bronchus (MA) there appear spot-like or patch-like whitening with definite border. A few patients may have whitish papula with lusterless surface, patch-like or strip-like prominence without obvious pressing pain. If chronic bronchitis is in the stage of acute attack, the area of Trachea (MA—IC2) may develop spot-like or patch-like whitening with flushed margin and lustrous surface.

Pneumonia: Spot-like or patch-like reddening or reddish papula with lustrous surface appear in the locus of Lung (MA—IC1).

Pulmonary emphysema: Patch-like or dense spot-like whitening with unclear margin in the locus of Lung (MA—IC1). If the disease is in the period of acute attack, the skin of the point locus become lustrous.

Pulmonary tuberculosis: In the area of Lung (MA — IC1) grey calcific spot of different sizes may appear, such as a millet-size one with lustrous surface or appearance of scar with uneven surface. If pulmonary tuberculosis is in the active stage, there may appear spot-like or patch- like congestion or papula with lustrous surface in the area of Lung (MA—IC1). If it is in the calcific stage, there may appear one or several needle-tip-size depressions, or patch-like dark grey with definite margin. As to cavernous pulmonary tuberculosis, the area of Lung (MA — IC1) may appear spot-like or patch-like dark red depression with lustrous surface in its center.

2. Gastrointestinal diseases

Acute gastritis: Spot-like or patch-like flush with lustrous surface and tenderness appear in the locus of Stomach (MA-IC).

Chronic gastritis: Patch-like whitening with unclear margin appears in the locus of Stomach (MA-IC). A few patients may demonstrate thickened skin and strip-like matter in the locus of Stomach (MA-IC). If chronic gastritis is in the stage of acute onset, the area of Stomach (MA-IC) may develop spot-like reddening in the patch-like whitening. An observation of 86 cases of chronic gastritis revealed that in the Stomach (MA-IC) area congestion was seen in 46 cases (53.5%), pale whitening in 37 cases (43%), and prominence in 61 cases (70.9%).

Gastric ulcer: Spot-like whitening or grey surrounded with definite flushed margin appear in the locus of Stomach (MA-IC). Remarkable tenderness is often found in the active stage while strip-like matter touched in the healing stage.

Chronic enteritis: Patch-like or congestive pupala with much grease appears in the loci of Large Intestine (MA-SC4) and Small Intestine (MA-SC2).

Acute hemorrhage of the upper digestive tract: Flush or congestion with lustrous surface appears in the corresponding area of the auricle.

Constipation: Patch-like whitening or furfuraceous desquamation with dull color appears in the loci of Large Intestine (MA-SC4) and Small Intestine (MA-SC2). Strip-like matter is palpable.

Appendicitis: In acute appendicitis, spot-like or papuloid congestion may appear in the locus of Appendix (MA-SC3), and blister-like flush in minority cases. In chronic appendicitis, spot-like depression or prominence may appear in the locus of Appendix (MA-SC3), and spot-like whitening or dark grey in minority cases.

3. Liver and gallbladder diseases

Hepatitis: In patients with acute hepatitis, patch-like or spot-like flush, or white-centered flush with lustrous surface and tenderness may be found in the locus of Liver (MA—SC5). In chronic hepatitis, patch-like whitening with spot-like flush in it, or patch-like prominence with spot- like flush or whitening in it may be seen in the locus of Liver (MA—SC5). A survey of 1300 healthy persons and 104 hepatitis patients shows that 4.7% of the healthy persons and 80.7% of the hepatitis patients had positive reactions in the locus of Liver (MA—SC5), with a remarkable difference between them ($P<0.01$).

Hepatocirrhosis: In the locus of Liver (MA—SC5), there may appear dense circular depressions with purple-brown color or prominence with definite margin and nodes inside, mild tenderness, and possible strip-like matters.

Cholecystitis: In acute cholecystitis, spot-like or patch-like flush with lustrous surface and obvious tenderness may appear in the locus of Gallbladder (MA—SC6), while in chronic cholecystitis, spot-like whitening with flushed margin and strip-like matters may present.

Cholelithiasis: About 85.5% of the patients have positive reactions in the locus of Gallbladder (MA—SC6). The commonly-seen are small nodes, spot-like whitening with definite margin, and strip-like matters which may has flushed margin and obvious tenderness when the disease is in the acute stage of onset. A report presents that 83.33% of the cholelithiasis patients had changes of skin color and shape in the locus of Gallbladder (MA—SC6), which was much higher than that of a control group consisting of healthy persons. Of the changes, the most commonly-seen was spot-like whitening (accounting for 90.74 % of the total), the numbers of which were associated with the numbers of the biliary stones. Moreover, the electric resistance of the center of the skin-changed area was lower than that of the surrounding normal skin.

4. Cardiovascular diseases

Hypertension: There may appear spot-like or patch-like flush in Central Rim (MA—AT), Subcortex (MA—AT1) and Adrenal

Gland (MA—T), folds in Heart (MA—IC), and spot-like whitening circled with flush in the upper one third of Lowering Blood Pressure Groove (MA). Appearance of strip-like substances in the Lowering Blood Pressure Groove (MA) is an indication of arteriosclerosis.

Hypotension: Spot-like whitening circled with flush appears in the lower 1/3 of Lowering Blood Pressure Groove (MA).

Coronary heart disease: About 71.31 % of the patients have positive reactions manifested mainly by color change of the area of Heart (MA—IC), mostly in red or dark red. In addition, a great majority of the patients with coronary heart disease have slanting folds in the ear lobe. It is reported that the dyeing rate in patients with coronary heart disease is much higher than that in persons without this disease. If unilateral dyeing is defined as positive, in the study group of coronary heart disease the dyeing rate was 91.7% and 80.0% in Heart (MA—IC) and Small Intestine (MA—SC2) respectively, while in the control group 25.0% and 20.0% respectively. There was a significant difference between the two group ($P<0.01$). If dyeing of bilateral Heart (MA—IC1) and Small Intestine (MA—SC2) simultaneously is defined as positive, then the dyeing rate was 78.3% and 3.3% in the coronary heart disease group and the control group, respectively. The difference was also significant between the two group ($P<0.01$).

Myocardiac infarction: In the acute stage, there may appear patch-like congestive flush in the locus of Heart (MA—IC), and dilation of microangium appearing in the congestive flush for minor cases. In the healing stage, spot-like or patch-like dark grey possibly with dark red or dark grey margin and depressed or prominent center may appear in the locus of Heart (MA—IC).

Pulmonary heart disease: Spot-like or patch-like whitening or flush in the loci of Heart (MA—IC) and Lung (MA—IC1), with bright surface in the attack stage and lusterless in the resting stage.

Rheumatic heart disease: In the locus of Heart (MA—IC), there may appear patch-like whitening with uneven surface and indefinite margin, angioplerosis and obvious tenderness.

Myocarditis: Scattered spot-like or papuloid congestion appears in the locus of Heart (MA—IC).

5. Urinary diseases

Nephritis: In acute nephritis, there may appear spot-like or patch-like flush with lustrous surface and obvious tenderness in the locus of Kidney (MA—SC), while in chronic nephritis, there may present patch-like whitening, or fold-like circle with lustrous surface, and papuloid whitening for minor cases.

Pyelonephritis: In the locus of Kidney (MA—SC), there may appear whitish papula, and patch-like whitening for minor cases.

Calculus of kidney: In the locus of Kidney (MA—SC), there may appear whitish papula circled with flush or spot-like dark red with definite margin.

Cystitis: In acute cystitis, the locus of Bladder (MA—SC8) may present spot-like or patch-like flush, or spot-like whitening circled with flush, and papuloid flush in minor cases. In chronic cystitis, there are spot-like or patch-like whitening, whitish papula, or folds with uneven surface and possible flushed margin in the locus of Bladder (MA—SC8).

6. Gynecological diseases

Annexitis, cervicitis and pelvic inflammation: Spot-like and patch-like papuloid flush with much grease in the surface appear in the locus of Internal Genitals (MA—TF).

Dysmenorrhea: Spot-like and patch-like papuloid whitening or flush with lustrous surface appear in the locus of Internal Genitals (MA—TF).

Amenorrhea: The locus of Internal Genitals (MA—TF) may appear spot-like and patch-like papuloid whitening with lusterless surface, and furfuraceous desquamation in minor cases.

7. Tumor

In the auricle, tumor is mostly reflected as nodular prominence and whitish streak in the corresponding area. In detail, the nodular prominence is usually movable and has clear margin and no pain or slight pain upon pressing in benign tumor patients while it is immovable and has indefinite margin in malignant tumor patients.

Liver cancer: The locus of Liver (MA—SC5) presents circular, elliptical or strip-like nodes with hard nature, or circular depressions arranged in the shape of plum flower with a skin color of light brown or dark brown.

Esophageal carcinoma: Nodular prominence and whitish streak with unclear margin or slight depression appear in the locus of Esophagus (MA — IC6). A report presents that diagnosis of esophageal carcinoma according to observation of the changes of shape, color and pain threshold in the loci of Esophagus (MA — IC6), Tumor-Distinctive Area1 (MA) and Tumor-Distinctive Area2 (MA) was identical to that of X-ray examination by the rate of 94.25%.

Gastric carcinoma: Nodular prominence of hard nature with unclear margin, obvious tenderness and rough skin may appear in the locus of Stomach (MA—IC). Positive being defined as milk-white or brown skin color and plum-flower-like depression in Stomach (MA—SC), an observation of 150 cases of stomach disease revealed that 22 of the 24 patients with positive reactions were confirmed to be carcinoma by pathological diagnosis while only one of the 123 patients with negative reaction was diagnosed as carcinoma. The remaining three patients with susceptible positive reaction were excluded from cancer by pathological examination.

Intestinal cancer: Node-like substance prominent to or level with the surrounding skin and obvious tenderness appear in the corresponding auricular points.

Lung cancer: Spot-like or patch-like dark grey with unclear margin and obvious tenderness appear in Lung (MA—IC1).

Hysteromyoma: Patch-like whitening and strip-like substance or circular node appear in Internal Genitals (MA—TF).

Recent achievements indicate a great significance of early diagnosis of tumor by auricular points. It is reported that 93.33% of the patients with primary liver cancer and 91% of the patients with hysteromyoma have positive reactions in the auricle.

8. Other diseases

Headache: There are spot-like flush with lustrous surface or whitish center, obvious tenderness and streak prominence in the antitragus.

· Arthritis: For chronic arthritis, spot-like or patch-like whitening with lusterless surface appears in corresponding auricular points. If in the attach stage, the whitening will have flushed margin and lustrous surface.

Hemorrhoid: Spot-like whitening with a reddening margin appears in the locus of Anus (MA—H5), and spot-like or patch-like dark grey in minor cases.

Neurodermatitis: Furfuraceous desquamation which is somewhat difficult to be wiped away appears in corresponding auricular points.

Seborrhea dermatitis: Seborrheic desquamation appears in the whole ear. Occasionally, patch-like flush with lustrous surface is seen.

The correspondence between the auricular points and disease is not the kind of one to one, and sometimes the reflection of auricular points is not specific. In another words, one auricular point may reflect a number of diseases, and one disease may be reflected in many a auricular point. Therefore, in order to improve the accuracy of diagnosis, the clinical information should be analyzed through arranging, summing up and contrasting according to the knowledge of Zang-Fu organs and Meridians in TCM and the knowledge of anatomy, physiology and pathology in Western medicine.

Though the auricular diagnostic theory is still immature, and the accurate rate of diagnosis by auricular points varies in different reports owing to individual experience and technique level, it is still greatly appreciated by medical workers and patients for its simple manipulation, absence of side effects, painlessness and low cost.

Auricular Treatment

Ⅰ. Indications and Contraindications

1. Indications

Auricular acupuncture has wide indications. Theoretically, auricular acupuncture can be applied to treat all diseases if used appropriately. In clinical practice, however, it may be excellently effective, markedly effective, mildly effective or even ineffective in treatment of different diseases. Therefore, it may be used as a sole, a chief, or only a supplementary therapy according to the condition of the disease. The author's experience shows that the following are the common diseases effectively treated with auricular acupuncture.

(1) Various pain syndromes: Having quite good analgesic effects, auricular acupuncture is extensively used to treat a variety of pain syndromes.

Nervous pain: Anginoneurotic headache, migraine, occipital neuralgia, trigeminal neuralgia, intercostal neuralgia, sciatica, etc.

Inflammatory pain: Pharyngolaryngitis, tonsillitis, herpetic keratitis, electric ophathalmitis, otitis media, periodontitis, parotitis, rheumatic and rheumatoid arthritis, mastitis, angitis, phlebitis, prostatitis, cystitis, pelvic inflammation, biliary colic due to cholecystitis and cholelithiasis, etc.

Traumatic pain: Sprain, contusion, stabbing wound, scald, fracture, dislocation, etc.

Postoperative pain: A variety of pain following operation, such as pain due to wound or scar.

Tumorous pain: Pain resulting from a variety of tumor.

(2) Inflammatory diseases: Acute conjunctivitis, keratitis, electric ophthalmitis, tarsadenitis, periodontitis, otitis media, tonsillitis, laryngopharyngitis, acute or chronic trachitis, pleuritis, mastitis, gastroenteritis, appendicitis, pelvic inflammation, orchitis, urocystitis, urethritis, cholecystitis, facial neuritis, etc.

(3) Allergic and collagen diseases: Allergic dermatosis, allergic rhinitis, allergic asthma, allergic colonitis, erythema nodosum, rheumatoid arthritis, urticaria, drug rash, etc.

(4) Endocrine diseases: hyperthyroidism, diabetes mellitus, diabetes insipidus, obesity, hyperprolactinemia, etc.

(5) Reproductive diseases: Irregular menstruation, dysmenorrhea, amenorrhea, climacteric syndrome, premenstrual syndrome, impotence, spermatorrhea, sexual hypofunction, infertility, etc.

(6) Infectious diseases: Auricular acupuncture has the function of subduing fever, relieving pain and enhancing immune function to improve recovery. Clinical observation has proven that auricular acupuncture is effective for such diseases as influenza, whooping cough, malaria, pulmonary tuberculosis, bacillary dysentery and infectious hepatitis.

(7) Other diseases: Neurosism, hysteria, dizziness, hypertension, arrhythmia, gastrointestinal dysfunction, chronic pain of waist and legs, cervical spondylopathy, retrograde affection of knee joint, chronic gastrointestinal disorder, sequelae of brain trauma, numbness of limbs. It is also often used for withdrawal from smoking and improving looks.

2. Contraindications

Although auricular acupuncture has no absolute contraindication, attention should be paid to the following conditions:

(1) For patients with severe heart disease, strong stimulating manipulations, such as electroacupuncture and bleeding therapy, are inappropriate.

(2) For patients with severe organic disease, such as severe anemia and hemophilia, auricular needling is contraindicated.

(3) Auricular needling is inappropriate for women with 30 days to 3 months gestation, and auricular acupuncture is forbidden for habitual aborter.

(4) Auricular needling should not be applied until some ear diseases such as ulcer, eczema and ulceration of frostbile are cured.

Ⅱ. Prescription of Auricular Points

1. Principles for selection of points

The principles of point selection are the theoretical basis of auricular point prescription in treating diseases. A rational selection of points is the key to the improvement of therapeutic effects. General principles are described as follows:

(1) According to corresponding area: It is the most commonly used and fundamental principle, according to which auricular points corresponding to the diseased are selected, e.g., Stomach (MA-IC) is selected for stomachache, Temple (MA-AT) for migraine, Sciatic Nerve (MA-AH7) for sciatica, and Lumbosacral Vertebrae (MA-AH) for lumbago. In Clinical treatment, the corresponding point is in most cases the primary point to be selected. Since disorder in a part of the body will reflect itself on the corresponding area of the auricle as tenderness, changes of skin color or shape, desquamation, or electric properties, the corresponding points are usually the reaction spots.

(2) According to the theory of Traditional Chinese Medicine:

Points are selected on the basis of Syndrome Differentiation, especially the Syndrome Differentiation of Zang-Fu organs and Meridians.

According to the theory of Zang-Fu organs, points are selected in terms of physiological functions and pathological manifestations of the Zang-Fu organs. For example, Lung (MA−IC1) is selected for the treatment of acne, urticaria and rhinitis because the Lung controls the skin and has its special opening in the nose; Kidney (MA−SC) for loss of hair, tinnitus and deafness because the Kidney has its manifestations in the hair and has its special opening in the ear; Heart (MA − IC) is selected for insomnia and dream-disturbed sleep, neurosis and schizophrenia because the Heart takes charge of mental activities; and Liver (MA−SC5) is selected for pseudomyopia, optic atrophy and glaucoma because the Liver has its special opening in the eye.

According to the theory of Channels and Collaterals, points are selected in terms of courses of Channels and Collaterals and their exterior-interior relations. For example, Bladder (MA−SC8) is selected for sciatica because the Bladder Channel runs the area the sciatic nerve supplies; Gallbladder (MA−SC5) is selected for migraine because the Gallbladder Channel is distributed in the lateral aspect of the head.

(3) According to the theory of Western medicine: Points are selected in terms of the knowledge of anatomy, physiology, pathology, etc. in Western medicine. For example, Subcortex (MA − AT1) is selected for the treatment of peptic ulcer because Western medicine considers that the development of ulcer is associated with overtaxing one brain, emotional disturbance, mental stress, worries, etc. Subcortex (MA−AT1) can regulate the cerebral cortical function to restore its action in regulating the secretion and peristalsis of the digestive tract. Sympathetic (MA−AH7) can also be selected for the treatment of peptic ulcer because over excitation of the vagus nerve is considered to be one of the causes leading to excessive secretion of the gastric acid.

(4) According to specific function of points: Points are selected in

terms of relatively specific function of the points. For example, Shenmen (MA—TF1) is a powerful point in relieving pain, it therefore is used for various pain syndromes. Ear Apex (MA—H6) is a relatively specific point in subsiding fever, lowering blood pressure, relieving inflammation and tranquilizing the mind, so it can be selected to treat fever, hypertension, insomnia and dream-disturbed sleep. Occiput (MA—AT) has the function of relieving dizziness, so it is used to treat Meniere's disease and motion sickness.

(5) According to clinical experience: Points are selected in terms of individual's clinical experience. The majority of auricular points are derived from clinical practice. Along with the application of auricular therapy, new points and new function of the previous points are successively found, which offers a new choice for point selection. For example, Angle of Superior Concha (MA—SC) is selected for the treatment of coronary heart disease, gastroduodenal ulcer and nasal hemorrhage, and Sympathetic (MA—AT7) is selected for the treatment of vascular diseases, such as thromboangiitis obliterans, phlebitis, aorto- arteritis and Raynaudi's disease. Experiment has revealed that stimulating Sympathetic (MM—AH7) can dilate blood vessels and ameliorate blood circulation and subsequently elevate temperature of limbs. Besides, Wind Stream (MA—SF) is selected for allergic diseases, Hepatitis (MA) for hepatitis, and Middle of Superior Concha (MA—SC) for ascites, all of which are examples of selection of points on the basis of experience.

The above principles of selecting points can be applied either separately or jointly. In clinical practice, consideration must be comprehensive, i. e., grasping the generality as well as the peculiarity of points, and selecting points on the basis of Syndrome Differentiation as well as clinical experience.

2. Methods for locating points

After points have been selected, accurately locating the points is essential for therapeutic effects. Different from the body points, auricular points has shapes of spot and non-spot. The great majority of auricular points are non-spot shaped or regional. Since auricular treatment is in most cases carried out by spot-like stimuli, determining the most favorite or sensitive stimulating spot in the point locus according to different condition and individual is of great significance for improving therapeutic effects. The following methods can be taken as references for locating auricular points.

(1) According to positive reactions: Positive reactions in point locus, such as changes of skin color and shape, desquamation, papula, congestion, and node, are selected as the stimulating spot.

(2) According to tenderness: The most obvious tenderness in point locus is selected as stimulating spot. Tenderness is the most common manifestation that disease reflect itself on the auricle, and the most obvious tender spot is usually the most effective spot for the disease.

(3) According to electric measurement: The favorite conductive point in the locus of auricular points, which can be detected with the help of auricular point detector, is selected as the stimulating spot. Auricular points are usually the low resistance points and that will become even lower when the corresponding part of the body is in disorder.

(4) According to auricular dyeing: The dyeing spot is selected as the stimulating spot.

Ⅲ. Treatment Methods

A proper treatment method is essential to therapeutic effects. Modern science and techniques have offered many means for choice in auricular treatment.

1. Filiform-needle-needling therapy

The filiform needle is adopted to puncture the auricular points to treat disease. This has been the most widely used method for stimulating auricular points. Suitable filiform needle is the non-disposable or disposable needle of 15 mm long and 0. 45—20 mm in diameter.

If the non-disposable needle is used, it should be sterilized strictly.

Procedure of puncturing

(1) Posture of the patient: Sitting is common. However, lying position is necessary for the first visit patient with nervousness, or those who are afraid of needling, badly ill, or generally weak.

(2) Sterilization: The auricle is susceptible to infection. If infection occurs, auricular chondritis may be caused. Therefore, when performing auricular acupuncture, sterilization should be more strict than that of body acupuncture. Routinely, the needle is sterilized with high temperature and pressure and the auricular points with 2% iodine tincture followed by 75% alcohol for deiodination. Different from body acupuncture, the sterilization of auricular points usually is applied to the whole auricle, either whole anterior surface or posterior surface.

(3) Insertion of needle: With the auricle fixed with the left hand (the middle finger supports the auricle at the opposite surface to help determine the depth of the insertion, and the needle is held with the right thumb and the index finger and inserted swiftly into the point. The technique of insertion may be rotating, thrusting, or combined use of both them. The angle of insertion is mostly perpendicular, and obliquely insertion (45° —60°) and horizontal insertion (15°) are applicable. The depth of insertion is dependent on the thickness of the patient's auricle. Generally, the tip of the needle reaches or goes into the cartilage but does not penetrate through it. Two to three millimeter is common for perpendicular insertion.

(4) Technique of manipulation: Rotating and lifting-pressing are frequently used. When performing rotating, hold the body of the needle with the lateral aspect of the index finger and abdominal aspect of the thumb, and rotate the needle with the movement of the index finger forwards and backwards in small extension. When performing lifting-pressing, hold the body of the needle with the abdominal aspect of the index finger and thumb, and do lifting-pressing movement. The lifting-pressing technique in auricular acupuncture is different from lifting-thrusting technique in body acupuncture. When performing lifting-pressing, the tip of the needle is

moved with the elastic tissues of the auricle to produce stimulation on the point, in fact, the tip of the needle is still in the same lay of the tissue.

(5) Sensation of needling: After manipulation, the patient should feel a sensation of pain, distention, soreness, numbness, hot, cold, or touching electricity. For sensitive subjects, a propagating sensation of Qi along Channels to a remote area or to the diseased focus may be elicited. For example, needling Gallbladder (MA—SC6) in cholelithiasis patients may elicit a needling sensation spreading along the Gallbladder Channel or presenting in the gallbladder area. The chapter *Jiu Zhen Shi Er Yuang* (Nine Needles and Twelve Yang-Primary Points) of *Ling Shu* (Miraculous Pivot)states that the essential of acupuncture is to obtain Qi, and therapeutic effects can be produced following arrival of Qi. The remark is also suitable for auricular acupuncture.

(6) Retention of needle: Thirty minutes is common for retention of needle. However, the time varies with different diseases. For patients with acute pain or strong constitution, the needle may be retained for a longer time (30—60 minutes), while for severe conditions or patients with weak constitution, it is retained for a shorter time (10—20 minutes). To strengthen needling sensation during retention of needle and improve therapeutic effects, the needle should be manipulated intermittently at intervals of five minutes.

(7) Withdrawal of needle: With the left hand fixing the auricle and the right hand holding the needle, the doctor pulls out the needle quickly, or first rotates the needle to the subcutaneous layer and then pulls it out quickly. After withdrawal of the needle, press the punctured point with dry cotton ball for a while to prevent bleeding.

(8) Course of treatment: Usually, auricular needling is performed daily with 7 — 10 sessions constituting one therapeutic course. After each course of treatment, discontinue the treatment for 5—7 days and then begin the next course.

Precautions

(1) For needling with filiform needles, 2—4 points is common in each treatment. Generally, unilateral points are treated with alter-

nate use of the two ears, or bilateral points are treated with alternate use of two groups of points.

(2) Strict sterilization is needed before performing needling.

(3) If the patient is in a condition of over hunger, over full, drunk, over fatigue, very weak after a severe disease, or over stress, auricular needling should not be given.

(4) Auricular needling is not suitable for women with less than five months pregnant.

(5) If there are frostbite, ulceration, infection, etc. in the location of auricular points, needling is forbidden.

2. Intradermal-needle-embedding therapy

The intradermal needle is embedded in the auricular points to treat diseases. This therapy can produce a persistent stimulation to the point, it therefore is particularly suitable for chronic diseases and various pain syndromes.

Procedure of embedding

(1) Sterilization: Intradermal needles and other materials used should be sterilized with high temperature and pressure method. Only soaking in 75% alcohol is inadequate for sterilization. The auricle or the auricular points are sterilized with 2% iodine tincture followed by deiodination with 75% alcohol.

(2) Embedding: Fix the auricle and stretch the skin of the point with the left hand, hold the mosquito forceps or homeostatic forceps with the right hand and grip a sterilized intradermal needle, and then insert the needle quickly into the selected auricular point. After insertion, the needle is fixed in the skin with the help of a small piece of adhesive plaster.

(3) Retention of needle: The embedded needle may be retained for about 3—4 days: shorter (1—2 days) in summer and longer (5—7 days) in winter. In order to enhance stimulation and improve therapeutic effects, the patient should be advised to press the embedded needle 2—3 times daily during retention of needle.

(4) Course of treatment: Generally, one therapeutic course consists of 5—7 treatments with an interval of 7—10 days between two

successive courses.

Precautions

(1) Points selected for each treatment should not be excessive (commonly 3—5 points), and the treatment is usually performed on unilateral points with alternate use of the bilateral points.

(2) During the period of retention of needle, the patient should avoid wetting the auricle to prevent infection.

(3) If severe distending pain develops in the needle-embedded area, which is possibly an indication of auricular infection, the embedded needles should be removed, followed by applying sterilization on the treating area. Antibiotic treatment can be given in case of obvious inflammation.

3. Seed-pressing therapy

Medicinal pills with smooth surface, plant seeds, or magnetic pellets are pressed on the auricular points with adhesive plaster. Seed-pressing is developed on the basis of needling and intradermal-needle-embedding therapy, and it has become the most popular method for its simple manipulation, safety, less sufferings and persistent stimulation to the point. Seed-embedding therapy can be used for various patients, especially suitable for the elderly people, generally weak patients, children and those afraid of needling.

Seeds commonly used

The following are frequently used: *Wang Bu Liu Xing* (Semen Vaccarae), *Huang Jing Zi* (Fructus Viticis Negundo), *Ji Xing Zi* (Semen Impatients), *Lai Fu Zi* (Semen Raphani), *Liu Shen Wan* (Six Miraculous Drugs Pill), *Hou Zhen Wan* (Relieving Sore Throat Pill) and magnetic pellet. Of them, vaccaria seed (Semen Vaccarae) and magnetic pellet are used most commonly. Compared with vaccaria seed, the magnetic pellet is more effective in tranquilizing the mind and relieving pain.

Procedure of pressing

(1) Sterilization: Seeds used for pressing are soaked in 75% alcohol for 2—3 hours after washed, and then dried in the air for later use. The auricle is sterilized with 75 % alcohol before treatment.

(2) Pressing: The seed is placed in the center of a small piece of adhesive plaster (the size of 0.5×0.5 cm) which is prepared previously. With the auricle fixed the left hand and a small forceps or curved mosquito forceps held with the right hand, the small piece of adhesive plaster stuck on the selected auricular point. After sticking, the seed is moved slightly until it is in the most pain-sensitive area and then pressed with steady pressure for minutes. Sometimes, to enhance stimulation to the point, another seed is stuck on the other surface of the auricle directly opposite to the point, and the two seeds are pressed oppositely.

(3) Retention of seeds: The stuck seeds can be retained for 3—5 days, shorter (2—3 days) in summer and longer (6—7 days) in winter. In order to enhance stimulation and improve therapeutic effects, ask the patient to press the stuck seeds 3—5 times daily during the period of retention of seeds.

(4) Course of treatment: For chronic diseases, the stuck seeds are renewed 1—2 times per week with alternate use of the two ears, and 1 course consists of 10 treatment sessions with an interval of ten days between courses. For acute diseases, this treatment can be given once per day with alternate use of the two ears, and 3—5 treatments constitute 1 therapeutic course.

Precautions

(1) Four to six points are appropriate in each treatment. Generally, in each treatment unilateral points are treated with alternate use of the bilateral points, or bilateral points are treated with alternate use of two groups of points.

(2) When one presses the stuck seeds, the force should not be too strong, and rubbing should not be performed to avoid injury to the skin and subsequently cause infection.

(3) If there is chilblain or inflammation in the selected points, seed-pressing can not be performed until it is cured.

4. Electroacupuncture therapy

Electroacupuncture is a combined therapy of needling with filiform needle and electric stimulation. Compared with single needling, electroacupuncture produces more strong stimulation to the points. In clinical practice, electroacupuncture is often used to treat cholecystitis, cholelithiasis, asthma, pain symptoms, arthritis, paralysis, etc.

Procedure of performing

(1) Needling: With the auricle fixed with the left hand (the middle finger supports the auricle at the opposite surface to the point to help determine the depth of insertion), the needle is held with the right thumb and index finger and inserted swiftly into the point.

(2) Connecting with electric stimulator: Commonly, the main point is connected to the negative electrode and the supplementary point to the positive electrode.

(3) Choice of waves: Generally, there are three kinds of waves available in an electric stimulator: successive wave, intermittent wave and dense-disperse wave. The low frequent successive wave produces excitative action on the nerves and muscles while the high frequent successive wave produces inhibitory action; the dense-disperse wave ameliorates local blood circulation and promotes recovery of the body function; and the intermittent wave excites the nerves and muscles, which is the most powerful wave in eliciting excitative efficacy.

(4) Adjustment of output: The intensity of output should be adjusted from weak to strong gradually. Intensity of output value varies with the tolerance of individuals. As a rule, small output is suitable for generally weak patients, children and those who are sensitive to acupuncture while big for strong patients.

(5) Course of treatment: Treatment is performed once daily with each treatment lasting for 15—30 minutes. One therapeutic course consists of 10 treatments with an interval of 5—10 days between courses.

Precautions

(1) Two to four points are proper for each treatment. If single point is used, the other electrode can be held by the patient or connected to another unrelated body point.

(2) The adjustment of output should be gradual from small to

big.

(3) During needle retention, needling sensation will decrease gradually because of adaptation of the body. Therefore, the output should be increased in time to maintain effective stimulation on the points.

5. Drug-injection therapy

A small amount of drug is injected into auricular points to treat diseases via stimulation on the points and pharmacological action of the drug. Drug-injection therapy is often used to treat facial paralysis, neurosism, headache, bronchial asthma, hypertension, pulmonary tuberculosis, toothache and gastrodeuodenal ulcer.

Drugs commonly used

(1) Herbal medicinal products: *Dan Shen Zhu She Ye* (Radix Salvae Miltiorrhizae Injection), *Dang Gui Zhu She Ye* (Radix Angelicae Sinensis Injection), *Huang Qi Zhu She Ye* (Rhiizoma Coptidis Injection), *Huang Lian Zhu She Ye* (Astragalus Injection), and *Ban Lan Gen Zhu She Ye* (Isatic Root Injection)

(2) Vitamin: Vitamin B_1 and vitamin B_{12}.

(3) Local anesthetics: Procaini hydrochloridium and lidocaini hydrochloridium.

(4) Sedatives: Phenobarbitalum and chlorpromazine hydrochloridum.

(5) Analgesics: Pethidini hydrochloridum, anadolum, and fortanodyn.

(6) Antiasthmatics: Adrendini hydrochloridum and aminophyllinum.

(7) Antispasmodics: Atropini sulfas and scopolamini hydrobromidum.

(8) Central stimulants: Lobelini hydrochloridum, nikethamidum, strychnini nitras, and securininum.

(9) Hormones: Hydrocortisonum and insulinum.

(10) Hemostatics: Adrenobazoni, salicylas, and vitamin K.

(11) Biological products: Placental tissue fluid and brain tissue fluid.

(12) Others: Normal saline and distilled water.

Procedure of injection

Two to three points are proper in each treatment. The auricle is sterilized routinely. A 1－2 ml syringe is used to draw 1 ml of medicinal solusion. With the left hand fixing the auricle and the right hand holding the syringe, the needle is inserted into the subcutaneous tissue of the auricle and each of the selected points is injected 0.1－0.3 ml of drug solution, gradually. After injection, a skin mound will appear in the treated point while the patient feels a distending pain or hot sensation in the auricle. Following injection, press the point with dry cotton ball slightly to prevent external permeating.

Treatment is usually started at the ear of the diseased side and then at the opposite ear, once daily or every other day, and ten treatments constitute one therapeutic course with an interval of 7－10 days between two successive treatment courses.

Precautions

(1) Aseptic manipulation is necessary to avoid infection.

(2) Drugs with strong stimulation should be avoided and corrosive drugs be forbidden.

(3) For drugs with a tendency to allergic reactions such as penicillin, they can not be used until intracutaneous test shows negative reaction.

6. Bleeding therapy

A therapeutic method conducted by pricking the auricular points with a filiform needle or three-edged needle, or by cutting them with a surgical knife blade to cause bleeding. Auricular bleeding therapy has the function of relieving inflammation, subsiding fever, tranquilizing the mind and stopping pain. In clinical practice, this therapy is often adopted to treat the following diseases: fever, tonsillitis, pharyngolaryngitis, hypertension, acute conjunctivitis, headache, trigeminal neuralgia, and sciatica.

Procedure of manipulation

(1) Kneading or rubbing: The purpose of kneading or rubbing is

to make the auricle congestion.

(2) Sterilization: Strict sterilization is necessary. Generally, the auricular point is sterilized with 2% iodine tincture followed by deiodination with 75% alcohol.

(3) Pricking or cutting: With the left hand fixing the auricle and the right hand holding the three-edged needle or filiform needle, the doctor pricks the selected point quickly, and then immediately squeezes the pricked point to bleed several drops. After bleeding, the wound is pressed with sterilized dry cotton ball for a while. If a surgical knife blade is used, the doctor can cut an incision of 0.5 cm deep to the dermas in the selected point. After bleeding, the incision is pressed with sterilized dry cotton ball for one day.

(4) Course of treatment: For pricking method, 4—5 points are selected in each treatment, alternating between the bilateral points. Five to seven treatments constitute one therapeutic course with an interval of 5—7 days between two courses. For cutting method, 2—4 points are selected in each treatment, alternating between the bilateral points. One therapeutic course consists of four treatments with an interval of 10—15 days between courses.

Precautions

(1) Kneading the auricle to make it congestive is important for successful bleeding.

(2) Aseptic manipulation should be performed and the patient is asked to avoid from wetting the wound in 24 hours after operation to prevent infection.

(3) This therapy is forbidden for patients with hemorrhagic diseases or those who have a tendency to beeding.

7. Magnetic therapy

Magnetic pellet or piece is stuck to auricular points to treat diseases via the magnetic influence on the auricular points. The magnetic intensity of the magnet ranges from 300 GS to 1500 GS, and the size of magnet should not be large. There are two principal methods used frequently: direct sticking method and indirect sticking method.

Functions and indications

Magnetic therapy has quite a good efficacy in tranquilizing the mind, relieving pain, itching and asthma, and improving sleep. Therefore, it is suitable for treating the following diseases: hypertension, headache, insomnia, tinnitus, deafness, allergic rhinitis, acute conjunctivitis, cough, asthma, urticaria, cutaneous pruritis, etc.

Manipulation

(1) Direct sticking method: The auricle is cleaned with 75% alcohol to remove grease. A magnetic pellet or piece is placed at the center of a small piece of adhesive tape and stuck to the selected point. If necessary, another one can be stuck on the opposite aspect of the auricle with their different magnetic polarities opposite each other, by which the magnetic force can be concentrated to penetrate the point and thus improve therapeutic effects.

(2) Indirect sticking method: A magnetic pellet is wrapt with thin absorbent cotton and then put at the center of a piece of adhesive tape, which is to be stuck on to the auricular point. In this way, the side effects resulting from the direct action of the magnet on the skin can be reduced.

(3) Course of treatment: In general, no more than four pellets are used in each treatment which lasts 3—5 days. Ten treatments constitute one therapeutic course with an interval of ten days between two courses.

Precautions

(1) During the period of treatment, a few patients may develop such adverse reactions as palpitation, dizziness, nausea, fatigue, drowsiness, a hot or itching sensation, blister and eccymosis in local area. Mild reactions will disappear spontaneously several minutes or days after treatment starts while severe reactions will disappear immediately after the pellets are removed.

(2) In the initial treatment, two points are appropriate to be chosen, no more than four points, because excessive magnetic pellets may result in interference of the magnetic field in each other and consequently affect therapeutic efficacy.

(3) For some chronic diseases, though the symptoms have disappeared or been improved in the following treatment, it is necessary to continue the treatment for a period of time to avoid recurrence.

(4) Discontinue the treatment whenever an allergic reaction presents.

Ⅳ. Treatment of Common Diseases

1. Acute tracheobronchitis

Acute tracheobronchitis refers to an acute inflammation of the tracheobronchial mucous as a result of infection of virus and bacteria, or allergic reaction due to physical or chemical irritation. Those who expose to cold, overwork, or experience a lower general or local defensive function are often affected.

Essentials of diagnosis

(1) Main symptoms are cough and expectoration. Initially, symptoms of the upper respiratory tract present, e.g., dry, itching and/or hot sensation in the throat, sneeze, nasal obstruction and running nose. When the trachea is affected, cough and expectoration will develop, and hemoptysis occasionally.

(2) General symptoms are mild, such as moderate fever (about 38℃), which will come down to normal in 2—3 days.

(3) Respiratory harshness and scattered rales.

(4) No obvious abnormality is found in blood test. When secondary infection occurs, the total leukocyte count increases.

(5) This disease should be differentiated from acute upper respiratory tract infection, influenza, measles and whooping cough. Upper respiratory tract infection has obvious symptoms of the nose and throat, but without cough and expectoration; and no abnormality is found in auscultation of the lungs. Influenza has a sudden onset, evident general symptoms, high fever, crepitant rales in the lungs, and increased leukocyte count. Measles and whooping cough have epidemicity and some special findings in laboratory examination, by which they can be distinguished from each other.

Treatment

(1) Prescription (Fig. 4—1):

Main points: Lung (MA—IC1), Trachea (MA—IC2), Adrenal Gland (MA—T).

Supplementary points: Shenmen (MA—TF1), Sympathetic (MA—AT7), Apex of Antitragus (MA—AT), Large Intestine (MA—SC4).

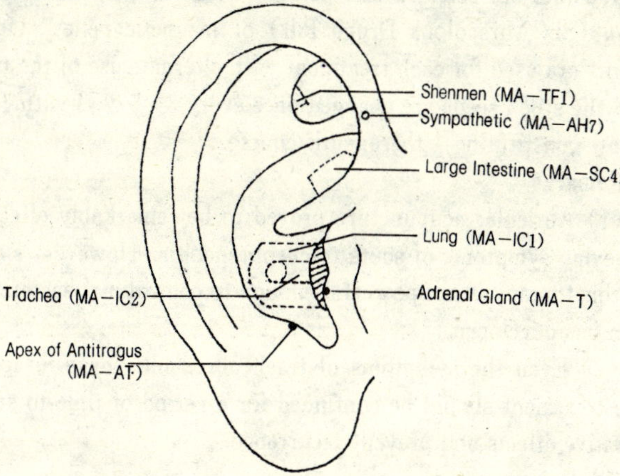

Fig. 4—1

(2) Methods:

Needling with filiform needle: In each treatment all the main points are used, and 1—2 of the supplementary points are added according to accompanying symptoms. After sterilization, needles are inserted into the points and manipulated with force every 5—10 minutes during 20—30 minutes' retention of the needle. The treatment can be performed once daily with alternate use of the two ears and 1 therapeutic course consists of 5 treatment sessions. For cases with severe cough, electroacupuncture may be combined to stimulate the main point and the successive wave is recommended.

Drug-injection: The commonly-selected drugs are *Ban Lan Gen Zhu She Ye*(Isatic Root Injection), *Chai Hu Zhu She Ye* (Radix Bupleuri Injection) and*Huang Lian Zhu She Ye* (Astragalus

Injection). If there is secondary bacterial infection, streptomycin or gentamicin may be used. Two of the main points and 1－2 of the supplementary points are selected in each treatment, and each is injected 0.1－0.4 ml of drug solution. The treatment is performed at the bilateral points once every other day and one course consists of three treatments.

Seed-pressing: All of the main points and 2－3 of the supplementary points are selected and pressed with vaccaria seed, *Liu Shen Wan* (Six Miraculous Drugs Pill) or magnetic pellet. Unilateral points are used for each treatment with alternate use of the two ears and the stuck seeds are changed once every 3－5 days with 10 treatments constituting 1 therapeutic course.

Remarks

(1) Auricular acupuncture proved to be remarkably effective for relieving symptoms of acute tracheobranchitis. However, single use of this therapy is not powerful enough to control it if bacterial infection has developed.

(2) Even the symptoms of tracheobranchitis have disappeared, the treatment should be continued for a period of time to stabilized curative effects and prevent recurrence.

Clinical reporte

It is reported that in patients with acute tracheobranchitis, congestion or spot-formed papuloid flush appeared in Trachea (MA－IC2), Lung (MA－IC1) and Pharynx and Larynx (MA－T3). Measurement of electric properties revealed that electrical resistance lowered obviously in the loci of Trachea (MA－IC2), Lung (MA－IC1), Antitragus (MA－AT) and Large Intestine (MA－SC4).

2. Chronic bronchitis

Chronic bronchitis refers to the chronic non-specific inflammation of the tracheobranchial mucous, and it is characterized by repeated attacks of cough and expectoration possibly accompanied with asthma. Chronic obstructive emphysema and even chronic pulmonary heart disease may complicate severe chronic bronchitis. Chronic bronchitis is a very common disease severely harmful to people's health. According to a survey, in China the incidence rate of chronic bronchitis is 3.83% of the population, and as many as 15% in the elderly people.

According to the patient's condition, chronic bronchitis can be divided into three stages: attack stage, delayed stage and remission stage. The attack stage refers to that excessive purulent or mucous sputum appears, accompanied with fever, or that any of cough, expectoration and asthma obviously aggravates within one week; The delayed stage refers to symptoms such as cough, expectoration and asthma at varying degrees lasting over 1 month; The remission stage refers to that symptoms have disappeared basically or that there are only slight symptoms such as cough and expectoration for over 2 months.

Essentials of diagnosis

(1) Productive cough, which become worse in the morning or in the evening, lasts for over 3 months or more in at least 2 successive years with absence of any other disease that might account for these symptoms. If there is objective examination evidence, diagnosis can also be established though the attack period is less than 3 months per year. Patients suffering from chronic bronchitis often has a long history of smoking or breathing in irritant gas or dust.

(2) Asthma and breathlessness, which are the chief manifestations of asthmatic bronchitis, and often attack in cold season.

(3) Repeated infection of the lower respiratory tract. When infection occurs, expectoration of purulent sputum presents.

(4) Auscultation of the lung finds normal or wet rales and wheeze.

Treatment

(1) Prescription (Fig. 4—2):

Main points: Lung (MA—IC1), Trachea (MA—IC2).

Supplementary points: Kidney (MA—SC), Adrenal Gland (MA—T), Apex of Antitragus (MA—AT), Shenmen (MA—TF1).

(2) Methods:

Needling with filiform needle: All of the main points and 1—2 of the supplementary points are selected in each treatment and punctured with 15 mm long needles. Strong manipulation is applied to the needles for patients in the attack stage while moderate for patients in the remission stage. The needles are retained for 20—30 minutes and manipulated every 5—10 minutes. The treatment can be given once daily with alternate use of the two ears and 10 treatments constitute 1 therapeutic course.

Seed-pressing: All of the main points and 3—5 of the supplementary points are selected. After the sensitive spot in the locus of the selected point is detected and cleaned with 75% alcohol, it is pressed with vaccaria seed or *Liu Shen Wan* (Six Miraculous Drugs Pill). Commonly, unilateral points are treated in each treatment with alternate use of the two ears. The stuck seeds are renewed once every 3—5 days with 1 therapeutic course consisting of 5—10 treatment sessions.

Intradermal-needle-embedding: In each treatment all of the main points and 1—2 of the supplementary points are selected and embedded with intradermal needle bilaterally. The needles are retained for 3—5 days with an interval of 2—3 days between 2 successive treatments. The treatment can also be applied at unilateral points with alternate use of the bilateral points.

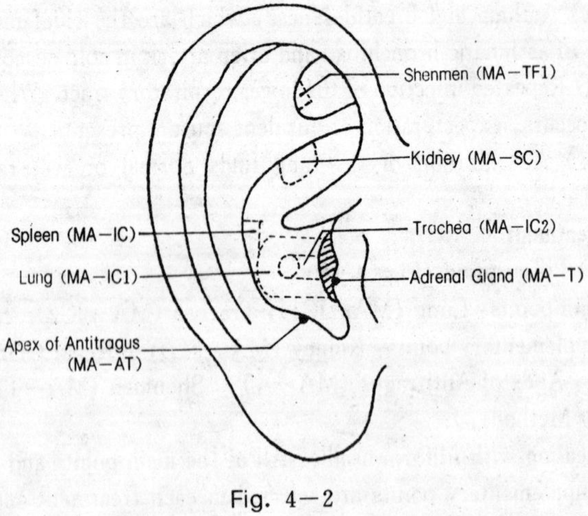

Fig. 4—2

Remarks

(1) For smoking patients, abstinence from smoking is essential for successful treatment, otherwise the obtained therapeutic effect will hardly be maintained.

(2) Chronic bronchitis, as a recurrent disease, takes the cough, asthma and sputum as Biao (the Incidental) and deficiency of the Lung, Spleen and Kidney as Ben (the Fundamental). Therefore, treatment should be given in attack stage and remission stage as well. By replenishing the internal organs to enhance the defensive ability of the body against disease is of important significance for eliminating this disease.

(3) During the stage of attack, needling with filiform needle at bilateral points is recommended, with alternate of two groups of points. During the stage of remission, however, seed-pressing and intradermal- needle-embedding at unilateral points are recommended, with alternate use of the two ears.

Clinical reports

(1) Zhang Hongshen et al reported 121 cases of chronic bronchitis treated with auricular acupuncture. Points selected were Shenmen (MA−TF1), Lung (MA−IC1), Adrenal Gland (MA−T) and Apex of Antitragus (MA−AT). If treatment lasted a rather long-term period, the above points were alternated with the following points: Subcortex (MA−AT1), Trachea (MA−IC2), Endocrine (MA−IC3), Pharynx and Larynx (MA−T3). Asthma Point (MA) or Sympathetic (MA−AT7) was added for severe asthma, Spleen (MA−SC) for excessive sputum, and Kidney (MA−SC) for elderly patients with weak constitution. Needling with filiform needles was performed, but intradermal-needle-embedding was given when long-term treatment was needed. Results: clinically controlled in 26 cases (21.5%), remarkably effective in 43 cases (35.5%), effective in 50 cases (41.7%), and ineffective in 2 cases (1.7%).

(2) Liu Xinlian et al reported 97 cases of chronic bronchitis treated with seed-pressing therapy. Points selected were Pharynx and Larynx (MA−T3), Trachea (MA−IC2), Lung (MA−IC1),

Large Intestine (MA－SC4), Kidney (MA－SC) and Endocrine (MA－IC3). Add Central Rim (MA－AT) for severe cough, Apex of Antitragus (MA－AT) for severe asthma, and Spleen (MA－SC) for profuse sputum. Vaccaria seeds were used for pressing. Results: clinically controlled in 30 cases (30.93%), effective in 54 cases (55.67%), and ineffective in 13 cases (13.7%). The total effective rate was 86.6%. Laboratory tests showed that seed-embedding improved the tests of phytohemagglutinin skin test (PHA), LTT and E-RFC at varying degrees, but could not improve IgG, IgA and IgM, indicating that seed-pressing can increase the ability of the body against infection but produce a little influence on humoral immunity.

(3) Deng Junping et al reported 100 cases of chronic bronchitis treated with seed-pressing therapy. Points selected were Lung (MA－IC1), Heart (MA－IC), Spleen (MA－SC), Kidney (MA－SC), Tonsil (MA－L), Endocrine (MA－IC3), Thoracic Vertebrae (MA－AH9), Shenmen (MA－TF1), Subcortex (MA－AT1), Central Rim (MA－AT), Sanjiao (MA－IC4), Lumbosacral Vertebrae (MA－AH) and Sympathetic (MA－AT7). Results: 45 cases were controlled basically, 47 cases were improved remarkably and 4 cases were improved mildly. The total effective rate was 96%.

3. Bronchial asthma

Bronchial asthma is defined as a disease characterized by an increased responsiveness of the trachea and bronchus to various stimuli, and manifested by widespread narrowing of the airways that changes in severity either spontaneously or as a result of treatment. Bronchial hyperactivity and reversibility of this trait are essential features. Asthma is characterized by such pathologic changes as hypertrophy of bronchial smooth muscle, mucous edema and hyperemia, thickening of epithelial basement membrane, hypertrophy of mucous glands, acute inflammation, and plugging of airways by thick, viscid mucus. These changes result in obstruction of airways of all calibers.

Asthma is common in adults and even more common in children. Men and women are equally affected. About 3% of the population has asthma. Death rates are increasing. A survey presents that the incidence of bronchial asthma is 0.5%—2.0% in China, However, there is also a report presenting an incidence of as many as 5.29%. About 20% of the patient has family history.

Essentials of diagnosis

(1) Recurrent episodes of asthma: Attacks occur spontaneously or result from various "trigger factors", including nonspecific irritants (dust, odors, fumes), emotional stress, infection, exertion, exposure to allergens, aspiration, and abrupt changes in weather.

(2) Sudden onset: Typical case is marked by expiratory dyspnea which reduces from several minutes to several hours followed by expectoration of excessive turbid sputum. Occasionally, dyspnea lasts for over 24 hours and the patient feels very difficult in breathing accompanied with dysphoria or disturbance of consciousness, excessive sweating and cyanosis, which indicates a critical condition called status asthmaticus.

(3) Wheeze: It is found in bilateral lungs in the stage of attack.

(4) Asthmatic bronchitis patients in most cases have years history of chronic bronchitis but no alternation of attack and remission, by which it can be differentiated from bronchial asthma.

Treatment

(1) Prescription (Fig. 4—3):

Main points: Lung (MA—IC1), Trachea (MA—IC2), Adrenal Gland (MA—T).

Supplementary points: Sympathetic (MA—AH7), Shenmen (MA—TF1), Superior Triangular Fossa (MA—TF), Endocrine (MA—IC3), Wind Stream (MA—SF).

(2) Methods:

Needling with filiform needle: This therapy is suitable for patients in the stage of acute attack. All of the main points and 2—3 of the supplementary points are selected bilaterally for each treatment. After sterilization, needles are punctured into the selected points and manipulated with force. The needles are retained until asthma is relieved. The treatment may be given once daily, or twice daily in severe cases. One therapeutic course consists of 5 sessions with an interval of 2—3 days between courses.

Drug-injection: The commonly-selected drugs are procaine and 1:1000 solution of adrenaline. According to the finding of detection, 2—3 sensitive points are selected bilaterally for each treatment and each is injected 0.1 ml of drug solution. This treatment is also suitable for patients in the attack stage.

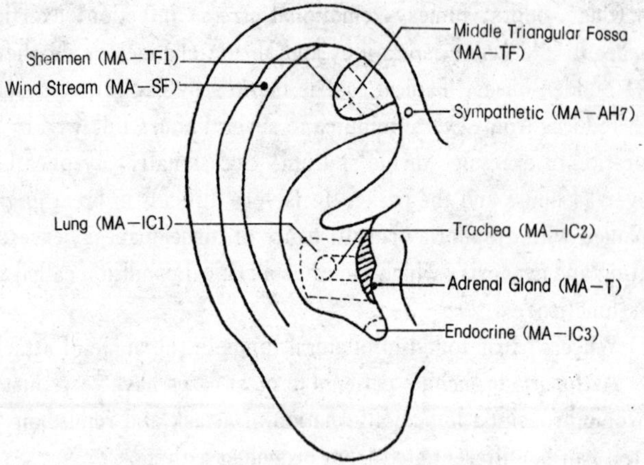

Fig. 4—3

Seed-pressing: This therapy is suitable for patients in the remission stage. All of the main points and 2—3 of the supplementary points are selected and pressed with magnetic pellet or vaccaria seed. Usually, in each treatment unilateral points are treated for mild cases with alternate use of the two ears while bilateral points are treated simultaneously for severe cases. The stuck seeds are changed every 3—5 days. One therapeutic course consists of 10 treatments with an interval of 3—5 days between courses.

Remarks

(1) Auricular acupuncture is effective for relieving asthma. However, to improve therapeutic effect, the patient should be asked to avoid contacting various anaphylactogen and do physical exercise to

prevent recurrence.

(2) Being a paroxysmal disease, asthma should be treated continuously for a period of time even though it has been relieved.

(3) For the patients of status asthmaticus, comprehensive management is necessary.

Clinical reports

(1) Wei Chijing et al reported 60 cases of bronchial asthma treated with pressing of vaccaria seed or *Bai Jie Zi* (Semen Sinapis Albae). Points selected were Trachea (MA－IC2), Lung (MA－IC1), Adrenal Gland (MA－T) and Angle of Superior Concha (MA－SC). Results: 31 cases were basically cured, 25 cases were improved remarkably, 1 case was improved mildly, and 3 cases were not improved. The total effective rate was 95%.

(2) Li Banglei et al reported 50 cases of bronchial asthma treated with auricular seed-pressing therapy. Points selected were Sympathetic (MA－AH7), Trachea (MA－IC2), Shenmen (MA－TF1), Kidney (MA－SC), Liver (MA－SC5), Spleen (MA－SC), Endocrine (MA－IC3), Adrenal Gland (MA－T), Bronchus (MA), Central Rim (MA－AT), Lung of Posterior Surface (MA－PS), Kidney of Posterior Surface (MA－PS), etc. Results: 42 cases were improved remarkably (84%), 6 cases were improved mildly (12%), and 2 cases were not improved (4%). Treatment sessions were 7 on average. Laboratory test revealed an obvious increase of hydrocortisone ($P<0.001$) after treatment.

(3) Zhao Zixiang reported 50 cases of asthma treated with auricular seed-pressing therapy. All of the patients suffered from recurrent attacks and failed to respond to antibiotics or presented drug resistance or allergic reactions. Points selected were: Sympathetic (MA－AH7), Shenmen (MA－TF1), Occiput (MA－AT), Central Rim (MA－AT), Lung (MA－IC1), Large Intestine (MA－SC4), Trachea (MA－IC2), Internal Nose (MA－T) and Kidney (MA－SC) as main points, Sanjiao (MA－SC3), Adrenal Gland (MA－T), Pharynx and Larynx (MA－T3) and Mouth (MA－IC5) as supplementary points. Vaccaria seed was used to press the points twice per week with alternate use of the two ears. For severe

cases, the bilateral points were treated simultaneously. The patients were asked to press the stuck seeds 3—4 times per day with each time lasting 5 minutes. Half a year's observation revealed that 12 cases were clinically controlled, 27 cases were remarkably improved, 10 cases were mildly improved, and 1 case was not improved. The total effective rate was 98%.

4. Chronic gastritis

Chronic gastritis refers to chronic inflammation of the gastric mucosa. Although the etiology of chronic gastritis remains unclear, it is considered to be related with bad habits, drinking, smoking, administration of irritant drugs, bacterial infection, bile-regurgitation, autoimmunity and some chronic diseases such as diabetes, hepatocirrhosis and hypothyroidism. Chronic gastritis is a common disease, especially occurring in middle-aged people.

According to different pathological changes, chronic gastritis can be simply divided into two types: superficial and atrophic. The superficial gastritis is characterized by congestion, edema and excessive mucus of the gastric mucosa, and scattered hemorrhagic spots and erosion may present sometimes; the atrophic gastritis is marked by pale and thin gastric mucosa and visible capillary network, and granular proliferation may be found occasionally. The two types have a close relationship and often exist at the same time.

Essentials of diagnosis

(1) Upper abdominal pain. It mostly appears in the upper abdomen below the xiphiod process and is characterized by dull, distending or stabbing pain without regularity.

(2) Dyspepsia. It is marked by abdominal distention, poor appetite, nausea and vomiting.

(3) Atrophic gastritis may present poor appetite, diarrhea, emaciation and anemia. Differentiation should be made between atrophic gastritis and stomach cancer.

(4) Fibergastroscopy and biopsy can not only establish diagnosis but also ascertain pathological nature: superficial or atrophic.

Treatment

(1) Prescription (Fig. 4—4):

Main points: Stomach (MA—IC), Sympathetic (MA—AH7), Shenmen (MA—TF1).

Supplementary points: Spleen (MA—IC), Liver (MA—SC5), Subcortex (MA—AT1), Pancreas and Gallbladder (MA—SC6).

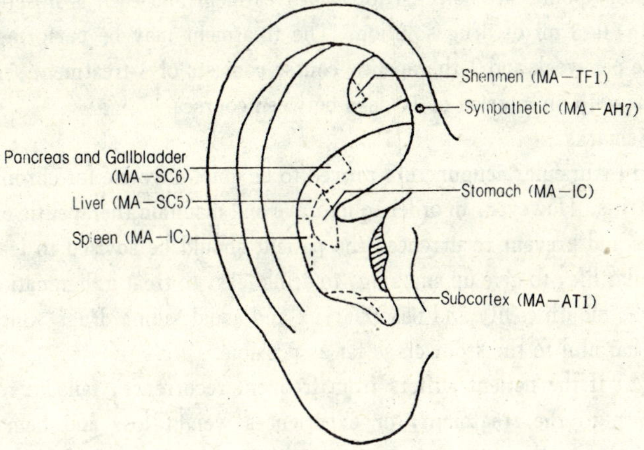

Fig. 4—4

(2) Methods:

Needling with filiform needle: This method is suitable for patients in the acute stage of attack. Two to three of the main points and 1—2 of the supplementary points are selected and punctured unilaterally in each treatment with alternate use of the two ears. According to TCM Syndrome Differentiation, the strong manipulation of the needle is applied to Excess type while the weak to Deficiency type. Needles are retained for 20—30 minutes. One therapeutic course consists of 10 treatment sessions with an interval of 10 days between courses. For Excess type, auricular electroacupuncture may be combined with needling.

Seed-pressing: All of the main points and 3—4 of the supplementary points are selected and pressed with vaccaria seed unilaterally in each treatment, alternating between the two ears. The stuck seeds may be changed once every 3—5 days and 1 therapeutic course consists of ten sessions with an interval of 3—5 days between courses.

Drug-injection: The commonly-selected drugs are vitamin B_1 and vitamin B_{12}, and *Dang Gui Zhu She Ye* (Radix Angelicae Sinensis Injection) and *Huang Qi Zhu She Ye* (Radix Astragali Injection) are applicable. Two to three of the main points and 1—2 of the supplementary points are selected for each treatment and each is injected 0.1—0.3 ml of drug solution. The treatment may be performed once per week and 1 therapeutic course consists of 4 treatment sessions with an interval of 10 days between courses.

Remarks

(1) Auricular acupuncture proved to be quite effective for chronic gastritis. However, in order to improve and maintain therapeutic effects and prevent recurrence, the patient should be advised to lead regular life, to give up smoking, to drink less, to treat inflammation of the mouth cavity and nasopharynx and avoid taking drugs which are harmful to the stomach as far as possible.

(2) If the patient suffers from frequent recurrence, fails to response to the treatment, or experiences weight loss and hematochezia, further examination should be given to ascertain whether cancerization occurs.

Clinical reports

(1) Sun Jingsheng reported 96 cases of superficial gastritis treated with seed-pressing therapy. Points selected were: Stomach (MA—IC), Spleen (MA—IC), Liver (MA—SC5), Sanjiao (MA—IC4) and Abdomen (MA—AH) as main points, Shenmen (MA—TF1) and Lung (MA—IC1) as supplementary points. After treatment, 56 cases recovered (58.3%), 28 cases improved remarkably (29.2%), 8 cases improved mildly (8.3%), and 4 cases failed to response (4.2%). The total effective rate was 95.8%.

(2) Wan Qihua et al reported 26 cases of chronic gastritis treated with auricular needling. Main points selected were Stomach (MA—IC), Subcortex (MA—AT1), Shenmen (MA—TF1) and Root of Vagus (MA—PS). Supplementary points were added according to Syndrome Differentiation: Liver (MA—SC5) and Spleen (MA—IC) were added for type of disturbance of the Stomach by the Liver Qi;

Small Intestine (MA－SC2) and Large Intestine (MA－SC4) for type of Deficiency of the Spleen and the Stomach; Spleen (MA－IC) and Ear Center (MA－H1) for type of insufficiency of the Stomach Yin; Spleen (MA－IC) and Pancreas and Gallbladder (MA－SC6) for type of incoordination between the Liver and the Spleen; Liver (MA－SC5) and Adrenal Gland (MA－T) for type of obstruction of the Stomach Channel; Esophagus (MA－IC6) and Cardia (MA－IC7) for type of internal impairment due to improper diet. Vaccaria seed was used to press the points. Results: cured in 8 cases, remarkable effective in 12 cases, mildly effective in 6 cases, and ineffective in 1 case.

(3) Wang Zhong et al reported 84 cases of gastritis either acute or chronic treated with auricular needling therapy. Main points selected were Stomach (MA－IC), Spleen (MA－IC), Sympathetic (MA－AH7) and Shenmen (MA－TF1), supplemented with Pancreas and Gallbladder (MA－SC6) and Liver (MA－SC5). Results: cured in 48 cases (57.1%), remarkably effective in 23 cases (27.4%), mildly effective in 7 cases (8.3%), and ineffective in 6 cases (7.1%). The total effective rate was 92.9%.

5. Gastroduodenal ulcer

Gastroduodenal ulcer refers to an acute or chronic benign ulceration occurring in the stomach and duodenum, clinically characterized by periodic rhythmical abdominal pain accompanied with acid regurgitation, belching and vomiting. Although the cause of gastroduodenal ulcer remains obscure, its onset is considered to be related with the following factors: heredity, bile-regurgitation, drinking of alcoholic beverage, smoking, administration of drugs harmful to the gastric mucosa, bad habits or life style, infection of pyloric bacillus, some endocrine diseases, and disturbance of gastric acid secretion due to dysfunction of the neurohumoral regularity. Gastroduodenal ulcer is a common disease and 10% of population are considered to have had this disease. It often affects young adults and has a delayed duration and frequent recurrence.

Essentials of diagnosis

(1) Long duration of disease, which ranges from several years to several decades.

(2) Regular recurrent upper abdominal pain, which is often induced by changes of season, over fatigue and improper diet but relieved by intake of food or alkaline drug. Each episode lasts for several days or several weeks. The nature of pain is indefinite: hungry sensation and/or hot pain in most cases and distention and stabbing pain possibly.

(3) Accompanying symptoms include nausea, vomiting, belching, acid- regurgitation, constipation, dyspepsia, etc.

Treatment

(1) Prescription (Fig. 4—5):

Main points: Stomach (MA — IC), Duodenum (MA — SC1), Sympathetic (MA—AH7), Shenmen (MA—TF1).

Supplementary points: Spleen (MA — IC), Liver (MA — SC5), Subcortex (MA — AT1), Endocrine (MA — IC3), Adrenal Gland (MA—T).

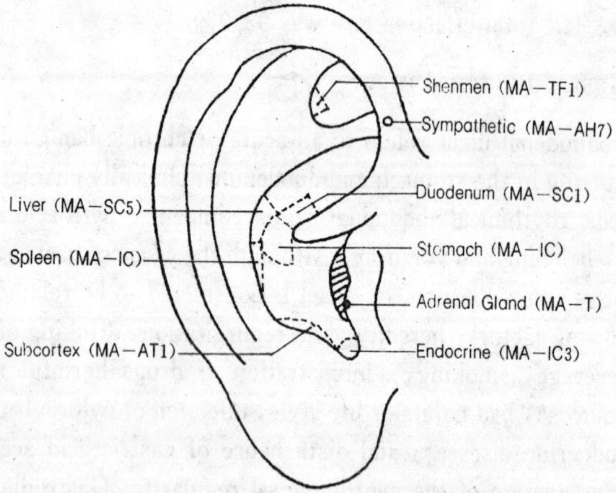

Fig. 4—5

(2) Methods:

Needling with filiform needle: This therapy is applied to patients who are in the stage of attack. In each treatment 2—3 of the main points and 2—3 of the supplementary points are selected and punctured unilaterally, alternating between the bilateral points. The choice of manipulations is based on TCM Syndrome Differentiation: strong pressing force for the Excess type while weak for the Deficiency type. Needles are retained for 20—30 minutes and manipulated every 5—10 minutes. The treatment may be given once daily and 10 sessions constitute 1 therapeutic course with an interval of 3—5 days between courses. For cases with obvious pain, combined use of auricular electroacupuncture can enhance analgesic afficacy, and the successive wave is recommended.

Seed-pressing: In each treatment 2—3 of the main points and 3—4 of the supplementary points are selected and pressed with vaccaria seed unilaterally with alternate use of the bilateral points. Strong pressing is applied to patients who are in the attack stage while weak to patients who are in the remission stage. The seeds are changed once every 3—5 days and 10 treatments constitute 1 therapeutic course with an interval of 3—5 days between courses.

Drug-injection: For patients in the stage of attack, procaine and atropine are recommended, while for patients in the stage of remission, vitamin B_1 and vitamin B_{12} are recommended. *Dang Gui Zhu She Ye* (Radix Angelicae Sinensis Injection), *Hang Qi Zhu She Ye* (Radix Astragali Injection) and *Dan Shen Zhu She Ye* (Radix Salvae Miltiorrhizae Injection) are applicable. In each treatment 2—3 of the main points and 1—2 of the supplementary points are selected bilaterally and each is injected 0.1—0.3 ml of drug solution. The treatment can be performed once per week and 4 treatments constitute 1 therapeutic course with an interval of 10 days between courses.

Intradermal-needle-embedding: In each treatment 1—2 of the main points and 2—3 of the supplementary points are selected and embedded with intradermal needle. Commonly the bilateral points are treated alternately. Needles are changed every 3—5 days and 7 times constitute 1 therapeutic course with an interval of 5—7 days between courses.

Remarks

(1) Pain relief does not mean complete recovery of ulcer. Therefore, treatment should be continued for a period of time after clinical symptoms disappear.

(2) Good habits and customs, proper life style and diet and a balance between work and rest are of important significance for stabilizing therapeutic effects and prevent recurrence. In addition, the patient should be advised to give up smoking and drinking and avoid drinking strong tea and coffee.

Clinical reports

(1) Wei Chijing reported 4 cases of gastric ulcer treated with seed- pressing therapy at Stomach (MA—IC), Adrenal Gland (MA—T) and Angle of Superior Concha (MA—SC). Symptoms were relieved in 1 case after 3 treatments, in 2 cases after 5 treatments, and in the remaining 1 case after 7 treatments.

(2) Prostaglandin (PG) can inhibit the gastric acid secretion to benefit recovery of ulcer. Laboratory test revealed that Angle of Superior Concha (MA—SC) can elicit the secretion of prostaglandin and consequently improve the restoration of the stomach function.

6. Hiccup

Hiccup refers to an involuntary, short, quick and frequent sound from the throat due to involuntary spasm of the unilateral or bilateral diaphragm. Hiccup may occurs in health persons due to quick swallow of dry food with rather small amount of water, which, however, may relieve spontaneously. It can also be a severe symptom developing in some diseases or following some abdominal operations.

Episodic phrenospasm may be caused by local stimuli to the phrenic nerve due to inflammation or tumor, stimuli to the vagus nerve resulting from diseases of the gallbladder, the stomach and other abdominal organs, or central nervous diseases such as inflammation and poisoning.

Essentials of diagnosis

(1) Paroxysmal hiccup with a frequency of several times to more than 20 times per minute, which in most cases can relieve itself.

(2) Functional hiccup and organic one should be differentiated. The former has no positive nervous sign while the latter usually has corresponding positive nervous signs.

Treatment

(1) Prescription (Fig. 4−6):

Main points: Ear Center (MA−H1), Root of Vagus (MA−PS), Stomach (MA−IC), Shenmen (MA−TF1).

Supplementary points: Sympathetic (MA − AH7), Subcortex (MA−AT1), Liver (MA−SC5).

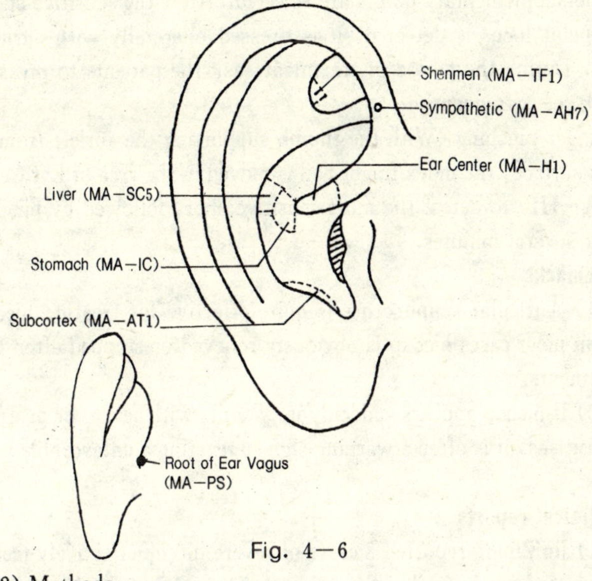

Fig. 4−6

(2) Methods:

Needling with filiform needle: In each treatment All of the main points and 1−2 of the supplementary points are selected bilaterally and punctured with filiform. The treatment can be given twice per day until it is relieved. The choice of manipulations is based on TCM Syndrome Differentiation: strong stimulating techniques for the Excess type while weak for the Deficiency type. Needles are retained for 20 − 30 minutes. Auricular electroacupuncture may be combined with it.

Intradermal-needle-embedding: Ear Center (MA—H1) and Stomach (MA—IC) are often selected. Fixing the auricle with the left hand and holding a filiform needle with the right hand, the doctor inserts the needle into Ear Center (MA—H1) obliquely and then pushs it forwards till the tip of the needle reaches the locus of Stomach (MA—IC). After manipulation of the needle with lifting-thrusting method, the needle hand is fixed to the skin with adhesive plaster and it is retained until hiccup is relieved.

Seed-pressing: in each treatment all of the main points and 2—3 of the supplementary points are selected. After the sensitive spot in the point locus is detected, it is pressed bilaterally with auricular seed. During the period of treatment, ask the patients to press the stuck seeds frequently.

Finger-pinching: With the thumb supporting the auricle from the back surface, the index finger nail is moved in the area of Ear Center (MA—H1) to detect the most sensitive spot, followed by pinching it for several minutes.

Remarks

(1) Auricular acupuncture is quite effective for treating hiccup, and in most cases hiccup is obviously relieved or stopped after 1—2 treatments.

(2) If hiccup appears suddenly in patients with severe or protracted diseases, it is often a warning sign suggesting a unfavorable prognosis.

Clinical reports

(1) Jin Ziping reported 8 cases of severe hiccup effectively treated with intradermal-needle-embedding therapy. All of the 8 cases were critical inpatients and had experienced other therapies without response. The duration of hiccup ranged from 18 hours to 5 days. Points selected were: Shenmen (MA—TF1), Ear Center (MA—H1), Sympathetic (MA—AH7), Stomach (MA—IC) and Subcortex (MA—AT1) as main points, Liver (MA—SC5), Kidney (MA—SC), Heart (MA—IC) and Large Intestine (MA—SC4) as supplementary points. Select four main points and 1—2 supplementary points in each treatment and embed cutaneous needles in them. Nee-

dles were retained for 3—5 days. During the period of needle retention, ask the patient to press the needles 2 times per day till needling sensation was produced. Results: 7 cases responded to the treatment and 1 failed to respond. 2 of the 7 responded patients had relapse, but both were relieved again after 1 treatment.

(2) Nie Hanyun et al reported 66 cases of hiccup treated with auricular acupuncture. Ear Center (MA—H1) was selected and punctured obliquely towards Stomach (MA—IC). The needle was manipulated with lifting-thrusting method to produce a strong aching pain, and hot or distending sensation, then it was fixed with adhesive plaster. Results: 64 cases recovered and 2 failed to respond. The time of treatment ranged from 2 to 48 hours in the cured patients.

(3) Gao Zhiying reported 16 cases of hiccup treated with auricular electroacupuncture. Points selected were Ear Center (MA—H1), Sympathetic (MA—AH7), Subcortex (MA—AT1), Spleen (MA—IC) and Stomach (MA—IC). The rapid successive wave (200 Hz) was applied and the output current was increased to the patient's maximal tolerance. The treatment was given daily with 1 time lasting for 30—60 minutes. All of the 16 cases were cured.

7. Ulcerative colitis

Ulcerative colitis, also called chronic nonspecific ulcerative colitis, is clinically characterized by diarrhea, mucopurulent bloody stool, tenesmus, poor appetite and emaciation. The etiology of this disease remains unclear, but it is generally considered to be related with autoimmunity, heredity, infection, food allergy and some neuropsychic factors. Pathological changes are manifested by recurrent inflammation and ulcer of the colon and rectum. Ulcerative colitis can affect people of all ages, more common in persons between ages of 20—50 years.

Essentials of diagnosis

(1) Diarrhea: The frequency ranges from 3—4 times daily to once 1—2 hours. The feces is usually sticky and mixed with mucus and purulent blood, but in severe condition it may consists of mucus and

purulent blood only. Occasionally, patients are marked by alternating between diarrhea and constipation.

(2) Abdominal pain: Commonly, there is a mild or moderate pain of colicky nature, which limits itself in the left lower abdomen or lower abdomen but sometimes involves the whole abdomen. Abdominal pain may be absent in mild cases. The pain may demonstrate a regularity of from abdominal pain to a desire to defecate, and then to pain relief following defecation.

(3) Delayed duration of illness and alternation of attack and remission.

(4) Feces examination finds erythrocytes, leukocytes and macrophages, but amebae are absent and bacillus dysenteriae culture is negative.

(5) Fibercolonoscope reveals that mucosa of the colon presents congestion, edema, a tendency to bleeding, small bleeding spots, and ulcers of different size and depth.

Treatment

(1) Prescription (Fig. 4—7):

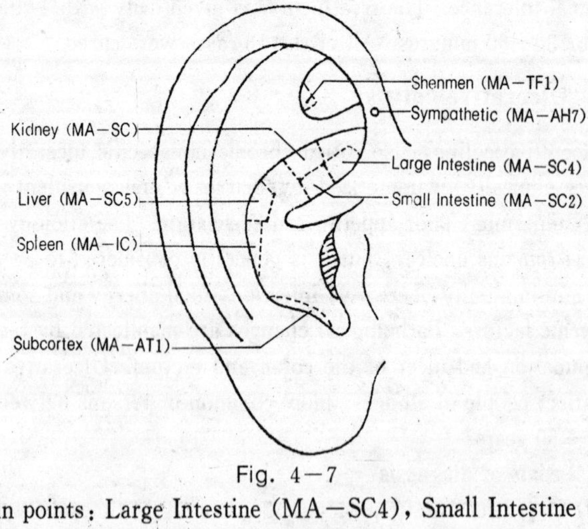

Fig. 4—7

Main points: Large Intestine (MA—SC4), Small Intestine (MA—SC2), Spleen (MA—IC), Sympathetic (MA—AH7).

Supplementary points: Liver (MA—SC5), Kidney (MA—SC),

Subcortex (MA—AT1), Shenmen (MA—TF1).

(2) Methods:

Seed-pressing: In each treatment 3—4 of the main points and 2—3 of the supplementary points are selected unilaterally and pressed with vaccaria seed or magnetic pellet. The suck seeds are changed once every 3—5 days with alternate use of the two ears. Ten treatments constitute 1 therapeutic course with an interval of 3—5 days between courses.

Needling with filiform needle: In each treatment 2—3 of the main points and 1—2 of the supplementary points are selected bilaterally and punctured with filiform needle once daily. The needles are retained for 20—30 minutes. Five to six treatments constitute 1 therapeutic course with an interval of 3—5 days between courses. This therapy is suitable for patients with obvious abdominal pain. After pain is relieved, seed-pressing therapy may be applied instead of needling to stabilize the therapeutic effects.

Clinical report

Cun Yunmeng reported 124 cases of chronic ulcerative colitis treated with seed-pressing therapy. Points selected were: Large Intestine (MA—SC4), Small Intestine (MA—SC2), Rectum (MA—H2), Liver (MA—SC5), Spleen (MA—IC) and Stomach (MA—IC) as main points, Pylorus (MA), Sympathetic (MA—AH7), Kidney (MA—SC) and Shenmen (MA—TF1) as supplementary points. Results: cured in 89 cases (71.8%), remarkably effective in 18 cases (14.5%), mildly effective in 10 cases (8.1%), and ineffective in 7 cases (5.6%). The total effective rate was 94.4%.

8. Constipation

Constipation, a common clinical symptom, refers to a morbid condition marked by decreased frequency of defecation and dry-hard stool with difficulty to be discharged. For healthy people, the frequency of bowels may be quite different because of different life style and dietary habit. However, most adults evacuate bowels once every day or every other day. If a person has not evacuated bowels for over 48 hours, accompanied with discomfort feeling, diagnosis of constipation can be made. The causes of constipation are various. It may result from organic diseases, such as partial intestinal obstruction, parenteral diseases which produce pressure to the intestine, anal fissure and disease of the spinal cord. It may also result from functional disorders, such as lack of intestinal dynamia due to old, general weakness and pregnancy, spastic colon, lack of food residue, administration of sedatives and antimelancholics, etc. Constipation discussed here chiefly refers to the functional one, and it can also be a reference for the treatment of organic one.

Essentials of diagnosis

(1) Dry and hard stool with difficulty to be discharged.

(2) The frequency of defecation is reduced to once every 2—3 days or even 5—7 days.

(3) Accompanying symptoms include abdominal pain or distention, headache, dizziness, anorexia, nausea, vomiting, palpitation and fatigue

Treatment

(1) Prescription (Fig. 4—8):

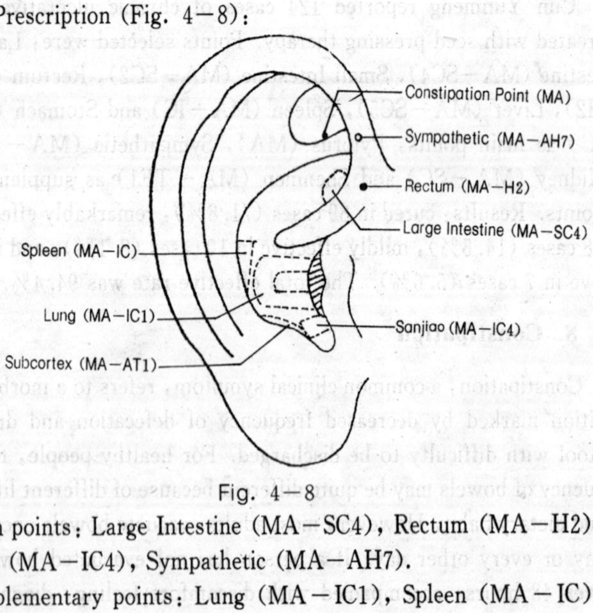

Fig. 4—8

Main points: Large Intestine (MA—SC4), Rectum (MA—H2), Sanjiao (MA—IC4), Sympathetic (MA—AH7).

Supplementary points: Lung (MA—IC1), Spleen (MA—IC),

Subcortex (MA—AT1), Constipation Point (MA).

(2) Methods:

Seed-pressing: In each treatment all of the main points and 2—3 of the supplementary points are selected unilaterally with alternate us of the two ears. Vaccaria seeds are used to press the selected points and they are changed once every 3—5 days. Ten treatments constitute 1 therapeutic course with an interval of 3—5 days between courses.

Intradermal-needle-embedding: Two to three of the main points and 1—2 of the supplementary points are selected. The treatment can be applied to the unilateral points once every 3—4 days with alternate the two ears or to the bilateral points with an interval of 2—3 days between 2 successive treatments. Ten treatments constitute 1 therapeutic course.

Needling with filiform needle: In each treatment 2—3 of the main points and 1—2 of the supplementary points are selected unilaterally with alternate use of the two ears and punctured with filiform needles. Needles are retained for 20—30 minutes and manipulated every 5 minutes, gental pressing for the Deficiency or atonic constipation while strong for the Excess or spastic constipation. Ten treatments constitute 1 therapeutic course.

Auricular electroacupuncture: In each treatment 1—2 of the main points and 1—2 of the supplementary points are selected and electrically stimulated. Usually, the intermittent wave is applied for the Deficiency type or atonic constipation while the slow successive wave or dense- disperse wave for the Excess type or spastic constipation. Needles are retained for 30—40 minutes. The treatment may be given at the unilateral points once daily, or every other day with alternate use of the two ears. Ten treatments constitute 1 therapeutic course.

Remarks

(1) Auricular acupuncture proved to be quite effective for treating constipation. However, to maintain therapeutic effects and prevent recurrence, the patients should be advised to eliminate induction factors and cultivate a good habits and customs, e. g., eating much

vegetables and fruit, especially those rich in coarse fiber, and drinking plenty of water. Sesame oil and honey are beneficial to defecation.

(2) For constipation occurring in patients suffering from acute cerebral vascular accident or paraplegia, other therapies such as cathartics should be given timely if the patients have no response to auricular acupuncture. If constipation results from intestinal obstruction, operation should be ready in case of failure of auricular acupuncture treatment.

Clinical reports

(1) Zhang Pingping reported 32 cases of constipation treated with seed-pressing therapy. Points selected were: Rectum (MA—H2), Large Intestine (MA—SC4) and Spleen (MA—IC) as main points, Sanjiao (MA—IC4), Small Intestine (MA—SC2) and Stomach (MA—IC) as supplementary points. Results: 21 cases were cured, 9 cases were improved, and 2 cases were ineffective. The total effective rate was 93.75%.

(2) Zhang Gengtian reported 33 cases of constipation treated with auricular needling. Main points selected were Constipation Point (MA) and Sympathetic (MA—AH7). Supplementary points were added based on TCM syndrome differentiation: Ear Apex (MA—H6) treated with bleeding therapy for Dry-Heat type, Liver (MA—SC5) for Qi stagnation type, Spleen (MA—IC) and Kidney (MA—SC) for Cold accumulation type, and Lung (MA—IC1) and Heart (MA—IC) for deficiency of Qi and Blood type. Constipation Point (MA) was punctured transversely forwards and the others obliquely or perpendicularly. Needles were retained for 40 minutes and rotated every 10 minutes. Treatment was given once every other day and a total of 3 successive treatments were performed. All of the 33 patients emptied their bowels following 1 treatment.

(3) Pan Jihua reported 134 cases of constipation treated with seed- pressing therapy. Main points selected were Large Intestine (MA—SC4), Constipation Point (MA), Spleen (MA—C) and Rectum (MA—H2). Supplementary points were added according to TCM Syndrome Differentiation: Ear Apex (MA—H6), Adrenal

Gland (MA−T) and Heat Point (MA) for Heat type, Liver (MA−SC5) and Sympathetic (MA−AH7) for Qi stagnation type, Kidney (MA−SC), Small Intestine (MA−SC2) and Spleen (MA−IC) for Deficiency type, and Kidney (MA−SC) and Adrenal Gland (MA−T) for Cold type. Three of the main points and 2 of the supplementary points were treated in each treatment. Vaccaria seeds were used to press the points and the patients were asked to press the stuck seeds 5 times daily with each time lasting for 4 minutes. Treatment was given every other day and 7 sessions constituted 1 therapeutic course. Results: 93 cases were cured, 29 improved remarkably, 7 improved mildly, and 5 were ineffective. The total effective rate was 96.3%. Comparing with a control group (n=80) treated with tab phenolphthaleinum, there was no significant difference between the total effective rates of the two groups. However, as regards to the cured rate and long-term effectiveness, auricular acupuncture was superior to tab phenolphthaleinum.

(4) Li Chengzhen reported 400 cases of constipation treated with seed-pressing therapy. Points selected were: Rectum (MA−H2), Large Intestine (MA−SC4) and Sympathetic (MA−AH7) as main points, Sanjiao (MA−IC4), Lung (MA−IC1) and Small Intestine (MA−SC2) as supplementary points. Results: 174 cases were remarkably improved (43.5%), 145 cases were moderately improved (36.25%), 62 cases were mildly improved (15.5%), and 19 cases were not improved (4.75%). The total effective rate was 95%.

9. Chronic cholecystitis

Chronic cholecystitis involves an inflammatory reaction of the gallbladder usually as a response to bacterial infection, chemical stimulation, or obstruction of the cystic duct. It is is the most common disease of the gallbladder disorders, characterized clinically by dull pain of the right upper abdomen, dyspepsia and aversion to greasy food. In most cases cholecystitis and cholelithiasis exist simultaneously. According to a survey, 90% of the cholecystitis patients suffer from cholelithiasis at the same time. Some patients develop chronic cholecystitis following acute one, but most of the patients have no history of acute cholecystitis.

Essentials of diagnosis

(1) Abdominal distention in varying degrees; abdominal pain located in the right upper abdomen or upper abdomen, which is usually a persistent dull pain radiating to the right scapular region. Biliary colic may be present in the stage of cute attack.

(2) Accompanying symptoms include hot sensation of the stomach, belching, nausea, vomiting and acid regurgitation. Fever may be seen in the acute stage of attack.

(3) Chronic cholecystitis may have no positive sign. If in the acute attack stage, tenderness or rebound tenderness may be found in the right upper quadrant, and occasionally the swollen gallbladder may be touched.

(4) Ultrasonic B examination reveals enlarged or reduced gallbladder with coarse and/or thickened wall and poor contraction. Cholelithiasis may be found.

(5) Cholecystography finds cholelithiasis and reduced or enlarged gallbladder with deformation and poor contraction.

Treatment

(1) Prescription (Fig. 4—9):

Main points: Liver (MA—SC5), Pancreas and Gallbladder (MA—SC6), Sympathetic (MA—AH7).

Supplementary points: Shenmen (MA—TF1), Root of Vagus (MA—PS), Endocrine (MA—IC3), Duodenum (MA—SC1).

(2) Methods:

Seed-pressing: In each treatment all of the main points and 2—3 of the supplementary points are selected unilaterally with alternate use of the two ears. Vaccaria seeds are used to press the selected points and they are changed once very 5—7 days. Ask the patients to press the stuck seeds 3—5 times daily during retention. One therapeutic course consists of 10 treatments with an inerim of 3—5 days between courses.

Needling with filiform needle: This therapy is suitable for patients in the stage of acute attack. In each treatment 2—3 of the main points and 1—2 of the supplementary points are selected bilaterally and punctured with strong stimulation techniques. Needles are retained for 30－45 minutes and manipulated every 5 minutes. The treatment may be given daily with 5 sessions as 1 therapeutic course. If biliary colic appears, combined use of auricular electroacupuncture can strength analgesic effectiveness.

Drug-injection: In each treatment all ofthe main points and 1－2 of the supplementary point are selected unilaterally, alternating between the two ears. Each point is injected 0.1－0.3 ml of vitamin B_{12} solution. The treatment may be given once every other days and 10 treatments constitute 1 therapeutic course. If the pain is severe, dolantin may be used for point injection.

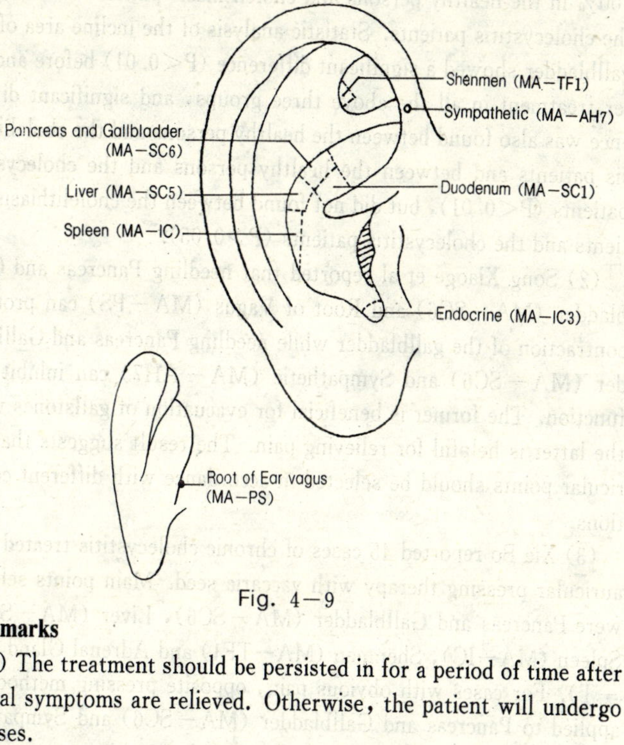

Fig. 4－9

Remarks

(1) The treatment should be persisted in for a period of time after clinical symptoms are relieved. Otherwise, the patient will undergo relapses.

(2) Advise the patient to take lower fat diet.

Clinical reports

(1) You Zhihong et al reported that auricular acupuncture can enhance contraction of the gallbladder. Subjects were divided into three groups: healthy persons (n=42), cholelithiasis patients (n=8) and cholecystitis patients (n=20). All of the patients were asked to keep in empty stomach in the morning before treatment. Auricular seed-pressing therapy with vaccaria seed was applied to bilateral Gallbladder (MA－SC6), Liver (MA－SC5), Duodenum (MA－SC1) and Sympathetic (MA－AH7). Ultrasonic B scan was performed before and at 30 minutes after treatment. Results revealed that after treatment the contraction rate of the gallbladder were 100% in the healthy persons and cholelithiasis patients and 95% in the cholecystitis patients. Statistic analysis of the incline area of the gallbladder showed a significant difference ($P<0.01$) before and after treatment in all the above three groups, and significant differerence was also found between the healthy persons and the cholelithiasis patients and between the healthy persons and the cholecystitis patients ($P<0.01$), but did not found between the cholelithiasis patients and the cholecystitis patients ($P>0.05$).

(2) Song Xiaoge et al reported that needling Pancreas and Gallbladder (MA－SC6) and Root of Vagus (MA－PS) can promote contraction of the gallbladder while needling Pancreas and Gallbladder (MA－SC6) and Sympathetic (MA－AH7) can inhibit this function. The former is beneficial for evacuation of gallstones while the latter is helpful for relieving pain. The result suggests that auricular points should be selected in accordance with different conditions.

(3) Xie Bo reported 45 cases of chronic cholecystitis treated with auricular pressing therapy with vaccaria seed. Main points selected were Pancreas and Gallbladder (MA－SC6), Liver (MA－SC5), Spleen (MA－IC), Shenmen (MA－TF1) and Adrenal Gland (MA－T). For cases with obvious pain, opposite pressing method was applied to Pancreas and Gallbladder (MA－SC6) and Sympathetic (MA－AH7) was added; for cases with vomiting, aversion to greasy food and poor appetite, opposite pressing method was applied

to Spleen (MA—IC) and Stomach (MA—IC) was added; for cases with obvious abdominal distention and diarrhea, Abdomen (MA—AH), Sanjiao (MA—IC3) and Small Intestine (MA—SC2) were added. Results: 9 cases were cured, 34 were improved, and 2 were ineffective.

(4) Wang Hongye et al reported that auricular seed-pressing therapy can thin the thickened gallbladder wall, elevate the ptosed gallbladder and change the arrangement of the gallstones, thus promoting the recovery of gallbladder function.

10. Cholelithiasis

Cholelithiasis refers to calculus existing in any part of the gallbladder and bile duct. Its etiology is still not very clear. Principal causes include accumulation of bile, bacterial or parasitic infection of the biliary tract and metabolic disorder of cholesterol. Cholelithiasis is a common disease and the incidence is 8.2%—14% according to a survey in China.

Gallstones can be classified as cholesterol calculus, brown calculus and black calculus. The cholesterol calculus, which often develops in a noninfectious gallbladder, contains about 60%—90% cholesterol, and the other two kinds of stones contain less than 40% cholesterol but much bilirubin.

Essentials of diagnosis

(1) Dyspepsia: Generally, patients are absent from symptoms or only have mild dyspeptic manifestations which become worse after a full meal or high fat meal.

(2) Biliary colic: The majority of the patients with calculi of the gallbladder have no biliary colic while those with calculus of the cystic duct and common bile duck may suffer from biliary colic which often attacks several hours after a full meal, high fat meal, or vibration of the abdomen.

(3) Physical examination finds tenderness or percussion pain in the right upper quadrant of the abdomen.

(4) Ultrasonic B scan can not only establish diagnosis, but also reveal the location, size and numbers of the stones, the severity of

pathological change of the gallbladder, and dilation of the common bile duct.

Treatment

(1) Prescription (Fig. 4—10):

Main points: Pancreas and Gallbladder (MA—SC6), Liver (MA—SC5), Duodenum (MA—SC1), Sympathetic (MA—AH7).

Supplementary points: Endocrine (MA—IC3), Shenmen (MA—TF1), Subcortex (MA—AT1), Small Intestine (MA—SC2), Root of Vagus (MA—PS).

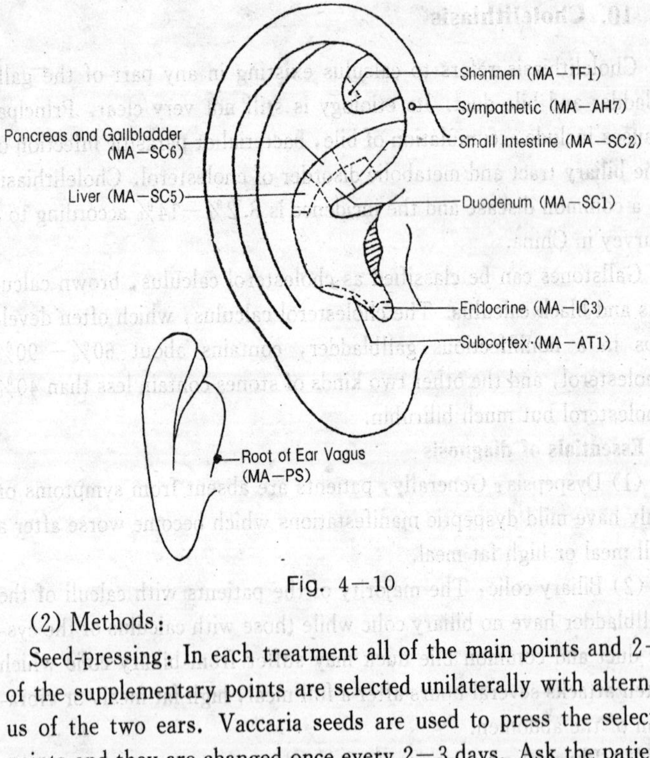

Fig. 4—10

(2) Methods:

Seed-pressing: In each treatment all of the main points and 2—3 of the supplementary points are selected unilaterally with alternate us of the two ears. Vaccaria seeds are used to press the selected points and they are changed once every 2—3 days. Ask the patients to press the stuck seeds 3—5 times daily. Ten treatments constitute one therapeutic course with an interval of 5—7 days between courses. To improve curative effect, detecting the most sensitive spot in the locus of the selected point is of great importance.

Auricular electroacupuncture: This therapy is especially suitable for patients with obvious biliary colic. Pancreas and Gallbladder (MA－SC6) and Root of Vagus (MA－PS) are frequently used. After needles are inserted into the points, they are electrically stimulated with an electric stimulator for 30－45 minutes. The treatment may be given once daily or every other day.

Remarks

(1) Cholelithiasis is one of the most common diseases being treated effectively with auricular acupuncture. Main points frequently selected are Liver (MA－SC5), Pancreas and Gallbladder (MA－SC6), Spleen (MA－IC) and Stomach (MA－IC), and supplementary points are added according to TCM Syndrome Differentiation or auricular detection.

(2) In the stage of attack, the patients should be advised to take high carbohydrate food but avoid fat diet; in the stage of remission, they should be asked to avoid high cholesterol food, such as animal brain, liver and kidney, fish and eggs.

Clinical reports

(1) According to a survey on cholelithiasis treated with auricular acupuncture, the rate of evacuation of gallstones is as high as 80%－90%, and the rate of complete evacuation of stones is about 20%.

(2) Li Zhanyuan et al have reported a comparative study. A total of 123 cases of cholelithiasis patients were classified randomly into four groups. ① Group A comprised 32 subjects treated with auricular seed-pressing therapy in combination with taking soup of pork's leg; ② Group B comprised 31 subjects treated with auricular seed-pressing alone; ③ Group C comprised 27 subjects treated with taking soup of pork's leg and placebo; ④ Group D comprised 33 subjects treated with taking placebo. Auricular pressing with vaccaria seed was applied to the following points: Pancreas and Gallbladder (MA－SC6), Duodenum (MA－SC1), Liver (MA－SC5), Stomach (MA－IC), Spleen (MA－IC), Large Intestine (MA－SC4), Rectum (MA－H2), Endocrine (MA－IC3), Sympathetic (MA－AH7), Adrenal Gland (MA－T), Sanjiao (MA－IC4), Small In-

testine (MA—SC2) and Root of Vagus (MA—PS). Results: in the group A, remarkable effect obtained in 9 cases (28.1%), moderate effect in 12 cases (37.5%), mild effect in 8 cases (25%), and no effect in 3 cases (9.4%); in the group B, recovery in 1 case (3.2%), remarkable effect in 10 cases (32.3%), moderate effect in 10 cases (32.3%), mild effect in 4 cases (12.9%), and no effect in 6 cases (19.4%); in the group C, remarkable effect in 4 cases (14.8%), moderate effect in 9 cases (33.3%), mild effect in 5 cases (18.5%), and no effect in 9 cases (33.3%); and in the group D, remarkable effect in 1 cases (3.0%), moderate effect in 10 cases (30.3%), mild effect in 5 cases (15.2%), and no effect in 17 cases (51.5%). Statistic analysis revealed a significant difference between the therapeutic effects of the group C and D ($P<0.001$), but no significant difference between the group A and B.

(3) Li Huifang et al conducted a study on the therapeutic efficacy of different seeds (plastic pellet and vaccaria seed) being used in auricular seed-pressing method in the treatment of cholelithiasis. Results revealed no significant difference between the two kinds of seeds ($P>0.05$), suggesting that the therapeutic effects produced by seed-pressing therapy are mainly resulted from the physical pressing rather than pharmacological properties.

11. Hypertension

Hypertension refers to an abnormal elevation of systolic pressure and diastolic pressure. The normal blood pressure is stipulated as systolic blood pressure $\leqslant$19 kPa and diastolic pressure $\leqslant$12 kPa. Hypertension is defined as the systolic pressure $\geqslant$21 kPa while the diastolic pressure $\geqslant$13 kPa, which are measured two times in different days. Hypertension is a common disease; according to a general survey of China in 1979, the incidence of hypertension was 3%—9% and it has a trend of increase. In the West, the incidence is as high as 10%.—20%. In about 90% of hypertension, no cause can be established. Generally, it is considered to be related with age, occupation, heredity and salt, etc.

Hypertension is classified as primary type and secondary type.

Those with unclear causes and chiefly manifested as elevated blood pressure is termed as primary hypertension while those as a clinical sign appearing in some diseases is termed as secondary or symptomatic one. Generally, so called hypertension refers to the primary type, and it is clinically manifested as pain and/or distending of the head, dizziness, palpitation, insomnia, blurred vision, and numbness of the extremities.

Essentials of diagnosis

(1) Critical hypertension is defined as the systolic blood pressure between 19 kPa and 21 kPa and the diastolic blood pressure between 12 kPa and 13 kPa; hypertension is defined as the systolic blood pressure ⩾ 21 kPa and the diastolic blood pressure ⩾ 13 kPa, which is measured twice in different days. When taking blood pressure, the patient should take a sitting posture and the right arm is measured.

(2) Clinically, hypertension is divided into three periods:

Period Ⅰ: Blood pressure has reach the level of hypertension, however, no complications of the heart, brain or kidney occur.

Period Ⅱ: Blood pressure has reach the level of hypertension, and at least one of the following abnormalities is found: ① Left ventricular dilatation detected by physical examination, X-ray, ECG, or ultrasonography; ② General or limited arteriostenosis revealed by examination of the optical funduse; and ③ Proteinuria and/or mild increase of the plasma creatinine.

Period Ⅲ: Blood pressure has reach the level of hypertension, and one or more of the following abnormalities is found: ① Cerebrovascular accident or hypertensive encephalopathy; ② Failure of the left heart; ③ Renal failure; and ④ Retinal hemorrhage or exudation with or without papilledema.

Treatment

(1) Prescription (Fig. 4—11):

Main points: Ear Apex (MA—H6), Groove of Posterior Surface (MA—PS), Kidney (MA—SC), Sympathetic (MA—AH7), Shenmen (MA—TF1).

Supplementary points: Heart (MA—IC), Kidney (MA—SC),

Subcortex (MA−AT1), Forehead (MA−AT), Occiput (MA−AT).

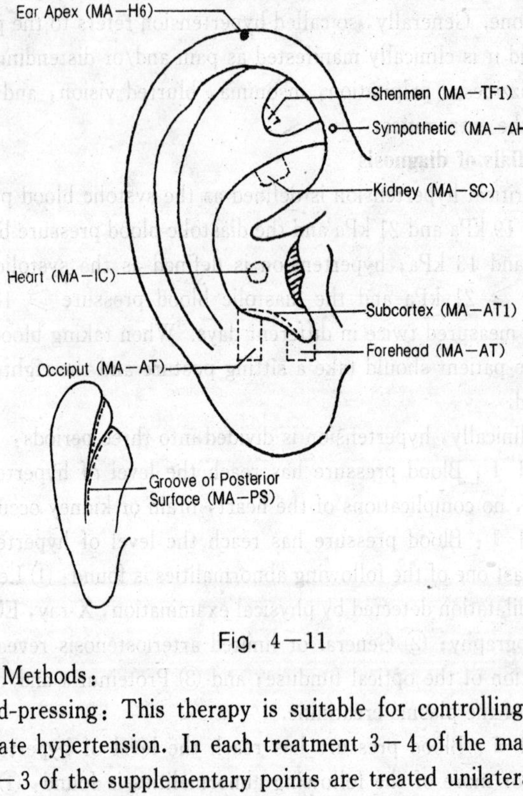

Fig. 4−11

(2) Methods:

Seed-pressing: This therapy is suitable for controlling mild or moderate hypertension. In each treatment 3−4 of the main points and 2−3 of the supplementary points are treated unilaterally with alternate use of the two ears. It is better to apply magnetic pellets. The stuck seeds are changed once every 2−3 days and 10 times constitute 1 therapeutic course with an interval of 3−5 days between courses. During seed retention, ask the patient to press the stuck seeds 3−5 times per day. Ear Apex (MA−H6) and Groove of Posterior Surface (MA−PS) may be treated with bleeding therapy.

Needling with filiform needle: It is better to apply bleeding therapy to Ear Apex (MA−H6) and Groove of Posterior Surface (MA−PS) and needling therapy to 2−3 of the other main points and 1−2 of the supplementary points. Needles are retained for 30—60 minutes. Manipulation techniques are performed according to TCM Syndrome Differentiation: strong stimulation for Excess type while weak for Deficiency type. The treatment can be given once daily or every other day and 10 sessions constitute 1 therapeutic course with an interval of 10 days between 2 successive courses.

Bleeding therapy: One of the small blood vessels on the posterior surface of the auricle is selected in each treatment. After kneading the vessel to cause congestion and applying routine sterilization, the doctor cuts it with a surgical knife blade to bleed 10 drops. Afterwards the wound is pressed with dry cotton ball and then covered with dressing. The treatment may be performed once every 5 days with alternate use of the 2 auricles and 4 treatments constitute 1 therapeutic course with an interval of 10—15 days between courses.

Remarks

(1) Pricking Ear Apex (MA—H6) to cause bleeding proved to be a simple and quite effective method for treating hypertension and the therapeutic effect is related with the amount of blood bleeded (5—10 drops in general). To bleed adequate blood, correct manipulation is important. According to the author's experience, the middle or posterior one third of the apex of the helix where Ear Apex (MA—H6) is located is selected as the treatment spot. After kneading or rubbing the area to make it congestive, the practioner pricks it quickly with a three-edged needle and then immediately squeezes its surroundings to facilitate bleeding.

(2) For hypertension, magnetic pellet is more effective than other kinds of seeds.

(3) Clinical observation shows that the therapeutic effect of auricular acupuncture is satisfactory for the treatment of period I and period Ⅱ hypertension. For the period Ⅲ hypertension, auricular acupuncture can improve symptoms but is inadequate to control the condition, internal management is therefore necessary.

Clinical reports

(1) Zhou Rongxing et al reported 135 cases of hypertension treated with auricular seed-pressing therapy. Vaccaria seed or medicinal

pill was used in the treatment. The medicinal pill was made by themselves, which consisted of *Zhu Ling* (Comprising Polyporus), *Ze Xie* (Rhizoma Alismatis), *Hong Hua* (Flos Carthami) and *Dan Shen* (Radix Salviae Miltiorrhizae). Points selected were Shenmen (MA－TF1), Sympathetic (MA－AH7), Liver (MA－SC5), Heart (MA－IC), Spleen (MA－IC), Kidney (MA－SC), Ear Apex (MA—H6), Helix 6 (MA—H), Subcortex (MA—AT1) and Groove of Posterior Surface (MA—PS). In each treatment, 5—6 of the above points were treated unilaterally with alternate use of the two ears. The seeds were renewed once every 3—4 days and the patients were asked to press the stuck seeds 5—6 times daily with each time lasting 5－10 minutes. Results: 61 cases improved remarkably, 30 improved, and 44 failed to respond. Both systolic pressure and diastolic pressure dropped significantly after treatment ($P<0.01$).

(2) Guan Zunxin et al reported 83 cases of hypertension treated with seed-pressing therapy. Points were selected according to TCM Syndrome Differentiation. ①For type of hyperactivity of the Liver Yang, Liver (MA—SC5), Kidney (MA—SC), Superior Triangular Fossa (MA—TF), Liver Yang (MA—H), Heart of Posterior Surface (MA—PS), Liver of Posterior Surface (MA—PS) and Kidney of Posterior Surface (MA—PS) are selected; ②For type of hyperactivity of the Liver Yang with deficiency of the Kidney Yin, Kidney (MA—SC), Sympathetic (MA—AH7), Subcortex (MA—AT1), Heart of Posterior Surface (MA—PS), Liver of Posterior Surface (MA—PS) and Kidney of Posterior Surface (MA—PS) are selected; ③For type of deficiency of both Yin and Yang, Heart (MA—IC), Kidney (MA—SC), Heart of Posterior Surface (MA—PS), Liver of Posterior Surface (MA—PS) and Kidney of Posterior Surface (MA—PS) are selected; And ④For type of accumulation of Turbidity and Phlegm, Spleen (MA－IC), Sanjiao (MA－IC4), Heart of Posterior Surface (MA—PS), Liver of Posterior Surface (MA—PS) and Kidney of Posterior Surface (MA—PS) are selected. *Cao Jue Ming* (Semen Cassia) was used to press the above points 3 times per week and 10 treatments constitute 1 therapeutic

course with an interval of 10—15 days between courses. Results: 12 cases were cured, 15 improved remarkably, 26 improved, and 3 failed to respond. The total effective rate was 85.5%.

(3) Liu Fuxin reported 103 cases of hypertension treated with auricular acupuncture. Main points used were Heart (MA—IC), Hepatitis Point (MA), Central Rim (MA—AT), Lowering Blood Pressure Point (MA). Supplementary points were added according to accompanying symptoms: Shenmen (MA—TF1) for insomnia, Gallbladder (MA—SC6) for dream-disturbed sleep, Heart Point (MA) for palpitation, corresponding points for the limb that was numb, and Ear Apex (MA—H6) for severe dizziness. Results: 85 cases were remarkably improved, 15 case were improved, and 15 cases were ineffective. The total effective rate was 95.7%.

(4) Tong Bing reported that electroacupuncture at either Ear Apex (MA—H6) or Lowering Blood Pressure Point (MA) were effective in lowering blood pressure. Statistic analysis showed the blood pressure significantly lowered after treatment and that Ear Apex (MA—H6) was more effective that Lowering Blood Pressure Point (MA) ($P<0.001$).

12. Ischemic heart disease

Ischemic heart disease refers to myocardial damage resulting from imbalance between the coronary blood supply and the need of the cardiac muscle circulation due to abnormal coronary circulation. It includes acute transient ischemia and chronic ischemia, caused by functional disorders or organic diseases. Those due to non-hemodynamic change of the coronary artery such as aortic stenosis are excluded. Ischemic heart disease can be classified into five types: asymptomatic type, stenocardia type, myocardiac infarction, heart failure and primary sudden cardiac arrest. Auricular acupuncture is suitable for the treatment of the first two types.

Essentials of diagnosis

(1) Asymptomatic type: Though clinical symptoms are absent, ischemia of the cardiac muscle is confirmed by subjective examinations, such as ECG, Load ECG and dynamic ECG. Coronary arteri-

ography finds obstructive change and biochemical index of insufficient blood supply. No histological changes are found in the cardiac muscle.

(2) Stenocardia type: It is characterized by paroxysmal retrosternal pain or precordial pain, but no histological changes are found in the cardiac muscle or only fibrosis is confirmed.

(3) Myocardiac infarction: It is characterized by persistent and severe stenocardia. Myocardial necrosis appears due to severe oxygen deficit and ischemia. ECG presents typical manifestations.

(4) Heart failure: It is manifested by failure of the heart, and cardiac dilatation and arrhythmia in the advanced stage.

(5) Primary sudden cardiac arrest: It is characterized by acute myocardial ischemia which leads to unsteady ECG and severe arrhythmia. Sudden death may be caused as a result.

Treatment

(1) Prescription (Fig. 4—12):

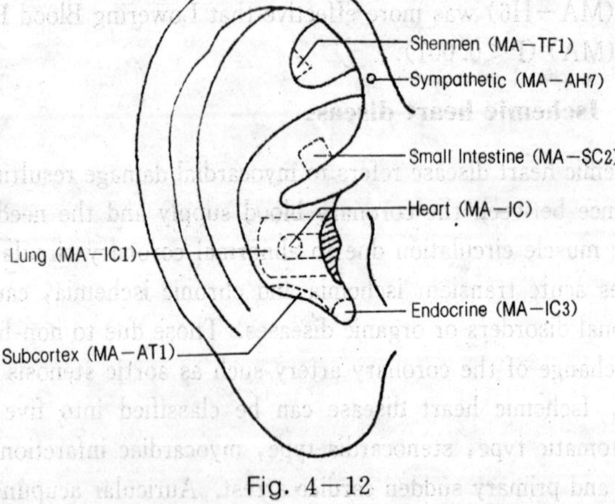

Fig. 4—12

Main points: Heart (MA—IC), Small Intestine (MA—SC2), Sympathetic (MA—AH7).

Supplementary points: Shenmen (MA—TF1), Subcortex (MA—AT1), Endocrine (MA—IC3), Lung (MA—IC1).

(2) Methods:

Needling with filiform needle: This therapy is suitable for those with aggravated symptoms and the stenocardia type. Needling is applied to all of the main points and 1—2 of the supplementary points bilaterally. The needles are retained for 20—30 minutes and manipulated with a strong stimulation technique. For patients with sternocardia, the treatment can be performed once or twice daily, while for those with mild symptoms, once every 2—3 days.

Intradermal-needle-embedding: In each treatment two of the main points and 2—3 of the supplementary points are selected and embedded with intradermal needles. For severe cases, bilateral points are treated simultaneously while for mild cases unilateral points are treated with alternate use of the two ears. Needles are retained for 3—4 days and the patients are asked to press the embedded needles 3—5 times daily.

Seed-pressing: In each treatment all of the main points and 2—3 of the supplementary points are selected, alternating between the two ears. If chest pain is obvious, it is better to use magnetic pellet. The stuck seeds are changed 2—3 times per week and 10 times constitute 1 therapeutic course with an interval of 3—5 days between courses. During the period of seed retention, ask the patients to press the stuck seeds 3—5 times per day.

Remarks

(1) Auricular acupuncture is quite effective in relieving symptoms of ischemic heart disease. However, improvement of ECG needs a rather long period of treatment (at least 3 months in general), and for advanced patients, single auricular acupuncture can hardly control the disease.

(2) Auricular acupuncture is suitable for chronic ischemic heart disease, and it can be used as a supplementary therapy for other kinds of heart diseases.

Clinical reports

(1) Wei Chijing reported 23 cases of coronary heart disease treated with auricular seed-pressing therapy. He used Heart (MA—IC), Posterior Coronary Artery (MA), Small Intestine (MA—SC2) and Angle of Superior Concha (MA—SC). Vaccaria seeds were used to

press the points and they were changed once every 6 days with alternate use of the bilateral points. During the period of retention of seeds, ask the patients to press the stuck seeds 4 times daily. Results: Symptoms disappeared and ECG restored to normal in 5 cases after 7 treatment sessions, and in 16 cases after 10 treatment sessions.

(2) It is reported that in patients with coronary heart disease, electroacupuncture at Heart (MA—IC) can improve myocardiac ischemia and regulate heart rate, which was manifested by normal or improved S-T period and T wave, reduced Q-X/Q-T ratio. Cardiac function was also improved, marked by reduced time before ejection of the left ventricle and increased time of left ventricular ejection. In contrast to Stomach (MA—IC) and Kidney (MA—SC), Heart (MA—IC) was relatively specific in association with the heart.

(3) Wang Lei et al reported 40 cases of ischemic heart disease treated with auricular seed-pressing therapy. Results: 16 cases recovered (40%), 20 improved (50%), and 4 failed to respond. The total effective rate was 90%. Patients with remarkable effects also exhibited an obvious improvement of EKG and restoration of ST-T.

13. Arrhythmia

Arrhythmia refers to abnormal heart beats, encountered in patients with heart disease as well as in healthy persons. Since some kinds of arrhythmia, such as slight sinus tachycardia and occasional premature beat, produce little damage to the body, medical management is not necessary. However, some kinds of severe arrhythmia, such as auricular fibrillation and ventricular tachycardia, can remarkably reduce the cardia output, so they should be given vigorous and effective management.

Essentials of diagnosis

(1) A detailed case history is very useful for diagnosis.

(2) Patients may have palpitation, dizziness, syncope, dyspnea, chest pain, etc.

(3) Auscultation of the heart may find tachycardia, bradycardia, arrhythmia and the inconsistency between the heart rate and the

pulse rate.

(4) EKG is of great value for establishing diagnosis.

Treatment

(1) Prescription (Fig. 4—13):

Main points: Heart (MA—IC), Sympathetic (MA—AH7), Shenmen (MA—TF1).

Supplementary points: Small Intestine (MA—SC2), Kidney (MA—SC), Root of Vagus (MA—PS), Subcortex (MA—AT1), Adrenal Gland (MA—T).

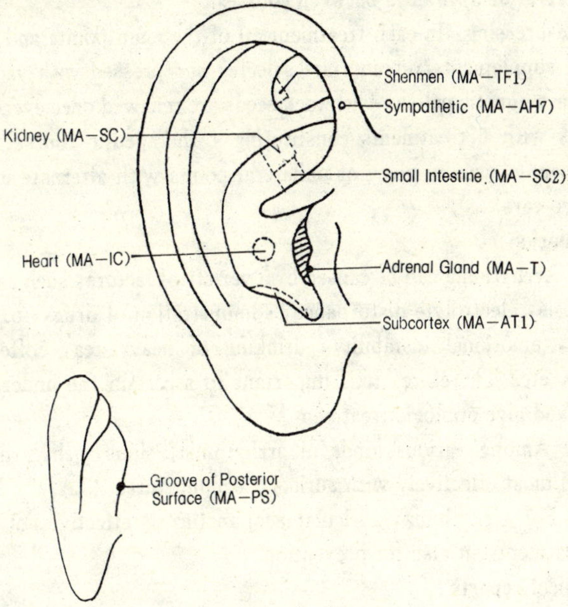

Fig. 4—13

(2) Methods:

Needling with filiform needle: This therapy is suitable for patients in the stage of attack. In each treatment all of the main points and 2—3 of the supplementary points are selected bilaterally. Needles are retained for 20—30 minutes and manipulated with a rather strong stimulation technique. The treatment may be given once daily and 10 sessions constitute 1 therapeutic course with an interval of 3—5 days between courses. If the disease is in the remission or stationary stage, the points can be treated unilaterally with alternate use of the two ears.

Intradermal-needle-embedding: In each treatment all of the main points and 1—2 of the supplementary points are selected and embedded with intradermal needles. The treatment is often applied to one side of the points with alternate use of the bilateral points. Needles are retained for 3—4 days and the patients are asked to press them 3—5 times daily. Five treatments constitute 1 therapeutic course with an interval of 3—5 days between courses.

Seed-pressing: In each treatment all of the main points and 3—4 of the supplementary points are selected and pressed with vaccaria seed or magnetic pellet. The stuck seeds are renewed once every 5—7 days with 5 treatments constituting 1 therapeutic course. The treatment is usually given at unilateral points with alternate use of the two ears.

Remarks

(1) Arrhythmia can be caused by a variety of factors, such as myocardosis, electrolyte disturbance, administration of drugs, oxygen deficit, emotional instability, drinking of heavy tea, coffee or liquor, etc. Therefore, it is important to ascertain the underlying cause and give etiologic treatment.

(2) Among various kinds of arrhythmia, sinus tachycardia is treated most effectively with auricular acupuncture.

(3) For arrhythmia, auricular acupuncture is effective not only for treatment but also for prevention.

Clinical reports

(1) Liang Jingwen reported 18 cases of supraventricular paroxysmal tachycardia treated with auricular needling at Heart (MA—IC), Shenmen (MA — TF1) and Sympathetic (MA — AH7). Needles were inserted to penetrate the auricular cartilage and left there for 30 minutes. During retention, needles were manipulated with moderate stimulation every 10 minutes. Treatment was given once every other day with 7 treatments constituting 1 therapeutic course. After 1—2 courses of treatment, all of the patients were cured, of which 5

cases were cured after 5 treatments, 9 after 1 course of treatment, and 5 after 2 courses of treatment.

(2) Wang Huilun reported that auricular seed-pressing therapy was effective for the treatment of arrhythmia subsequent to myocarditis. Points selected were: Heart (MA−IC), Small Intestine (MA−SC2), Kidney (MA−SC), Angle of Superior Concha (MA−SC) and Moderate−Small Arteries (MA) for atrial, ventricle or atrioventricular extrasystole; Atrioventricular Node (MA), Adrenal Gland (MA−T) and Vagus Nerve (MA) for the first degree A−V block. *Yan Hou Wan* (Throat Pill) or vaccaria seeds were used to press the points bilaterally and they were changed once every 3−5 days with ten treatments constituting one therapeutic course. After treatment, all patients were cured, of which one patient recovered within half a course of treatment, nine after one course, two after one and a half courses, and one after two courses.

(3) Li Shuping reported 34 cases of tachycardia treated by auricular pressing therapy with vaccaria seed, of which 30 were sinus tachycardia and 4 were supraventricular tachycardia. Points selected were Heart (MA−IC), Mouth (MA−IC5), Small Intestine (MA−SC2), Shenmen (MA−TF1), Sanjiao (MA−IC4) and positive reaction spots. Of the 34 patients with sinus tachycardia, 30 were improved remarkably, 6 were improved and 2 were not improved. The total effective rate was 93.3%. However, all of the four patients with supraventricular tachycardia failed to respond. The author of this article pointed out that stimulating auricular points can excite the vagus nerve and subsequently slow down the heart rate.

14. Migraine

Classic migraine headache is a lateralized throbbing headache that occurs episodically following its onset in adolescence or early adult life. In many cases, however, the headache may present as other manifestations, although their associated features and response to antimigrainous preparations nevertheless suggest that they have a similar basis. In this broader sense, migrainous headaches may be lateralized or generalized, dull or throbbing, and is sometimes associated with anorexia, nausea, vomiting, photophobia, and blurring of vision.

About half of the patients have a family history of migraine, and females are affected more often than males. Although the etiology of this disease remains unknown, it is considered to be related with heredity, endocrine dysfunction, emotional factors, etc. During the process of onset, initially contraction of the intracranial arteries brings about premonitory symptoms, then dilation of the intracranial and extracranial arteries and reduced pain threshold result in headache.

Essentials of diagnosis

(1) Headache often triggered by fatigue, stress, emotional instability, poor sleep, missed meals, specific food (e.g., chocolate and milk products), alcoholic beverages, menstruation or in a special season.

(2) Some patients have premonitory symptoms, such as blurred vision, aversion to light, flash point, blind spot, hemianopsia, distending pain of the eye ball, general discomfort, aphasia, numbness of fingers and lips, and dizziness. However, the most common symptom is visual abnormality.

(3) Pain is usually limited to the unilateral forehead, temporal region or orbit, and a few patients have bilateral pain.

(4) It may be accompanied with gastrointestinal and vegetative nerve symptoms, such as nausea, vomiting, abdominal distention, diarrhea, profuse perspiration, lacrimation, pale complexion, purplish skin with edema, and tachycardia or bradycardia.

(5) Most patients have a family history of migraine.

Treatment

(1) Prescription (Fig. 4—14):

Main points: Shenmen (MA—TF1), Subcortex (MA—AT1), Temple (MA—AT), Sympathetic (MA—AH7).

Supplementary points: Liver (MA—SC5), Gallbladder (MA—SC6), Ear Apex (MA—H6), Heart (MA—IC).

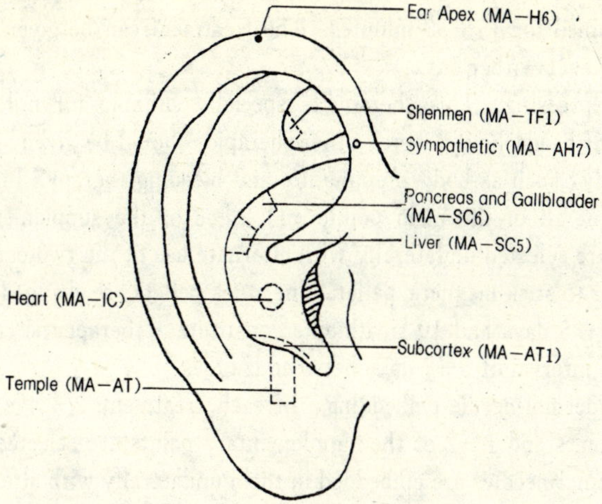

Fig. 4—14

(2) Methods:

Needling with filiform needle: This therapy is suitable for patients in the stage of attack. In each treatment 2—3 of the main points and 1—2 of the supplementary points are selected bilaterally and punctured with filiform needle. The needles are retained for 30—45 minutes and manipulated with a strong stimulation technique. The treatment can be given once daily and 5 sessions constitute 1 therapeutic course with an interval of 2—3 days between courses. If migraine is in the remission or stationary stage, it is recommended to puncture the points unilaterally, alternating between the two ears.

Electroacupuncture: This therapy is suitable for patients in the acute stage of attack. In each treatment 1—2 of the main points and 1—2 of the supplementary points are selected. After insertion of the needle, the points are stimulated electrically with an electric stimulator. The index of stimulation are selected and adjusted according to TCM Syndrome Differentiation and the patient's tolerance. For Excess type, successive wave or dense-disperse wave is recommended with an output maximal to the patient's tolerance, and the needles are retained for 30—40 minutes. For Deficiency type, intermittent wave is recommended with a moderate output, and the needles are retained for 15—30 minutes. The treatment can be given once daily or every other day.

Seed-pressing: This therapy is specially suitable for mild patients. If headache is severe, other therapies should be given simultaneously, such as body acupuncture and bleeding therapy. In each treatment all of the main points and 2—3 of the supplementary points are selected unilaterally with alternate use of the two ears. It is better to stick magnetic pellet. The stuck pellets are changed once every 3—5 days and 10 treatments constitute 1 therapeutic course with an interval of 5—7 days between courses.

Intradermal-needle-embedding: In each treatment 2—4 of the main points and 1—2 of the supplementary points are selected and intradermal needles are embedded in them unilaterally with alternate use of the two ears. The needles are retained for 3—4 days and the patient is asked to press them 3—5 times daily. Five treatments constitute 1 therapeutic course with an interval of 3—5 days between courses.

Bleeding therapy: This is one of the most effective therapies, especially suitable for severe headache or the Excess type. In each treatment all of the main points and 1—2 of the supplementary points are selected. First knead the auricle to make it congestive and apply routine sterilization, then cut the selected points with a surgical blade to bleed 1—2 drops for each point. After bleedling, clear away blood stain with sterilized dry cotton ball and cover them with dressing. Usually, the ear on the diseased side is treated firstly, and the opposite ear secondly. The treatment can be given once every other day and 2 sessions constitute 1 therapeutic course with an interval of 7 days between courses.

Remarks

(1) Auricular acupuncture proved to be quite effective for treating migraine, especially auricular bleeding therapy. According to the author's experience, headache is often relieved immediately following treatment.

(2) The etiology and mechanism of migraine are complicated, involving society, psychology and biology. It is closely associated with

diet and life habits and customs. Therefore, the patients should be advised to pay attention to their life style and eating habits. According to clinical observation and research, the following food are harmful to migraineur: milk products, fruit rich in citric acid, banana, walnut, chocolate and monosodium glutamate.

Clinical reports

(1) Lai Xinping reported 128 cases of nervous headache treated with auricular seed-pressing with vaccaria seed. Points selected were Liver (MA—SC5), Kidney (MA—SC), Central Rim (MA—AT), Shenmen (MA—TF1) and Subcortex (MA—AT1). Treatment was performed at the above points once every other day with alternate use of the two ears. During treatment, the patients were asked to press the stuck seeds to cause the auricle to be flushed and hot 3 — 5 times daily. Five treatments constituted 1 therapeutic course. Results: 57 cases recovered, 25 improved remarkably, 32 improved, and 4 failed to respond. In a control group (n=30) treated with oral administration of *Qu Tong Pian* (Relieving Pain Tablet), oryzanol and vitamin B_1, 10 case were cured, 7 were remarkably improved, 8 were improved, and 5 were not improved. Statistic analysis of the effective rate in the two groups revealed a significant difference in favor of the auricular acupuncture therapy ($P<0.05$).

(2) Sun Xiuben reported that bloodletting on the posterior aspect of the auricle is relatively good effective for angioneurotic headache. There are three obvious vessels in the upper one third portion of the posterior surface of the surgical, of which the mildde one is most suitable. In each treatment unilateral vessel was treated for migraine while bilateral for pain of the whole headache. First knead the auricle to make it to be congested and apply routine sterilization, then prick the vessel with a three-edged needle or cut it with a small surgical blade to bleed approximately 5 ml. The treatment was performed once every 15 days and 5 treatments constituted 1 therapeutic course. Of the total 120 cases observed, 74 were cured (no recurrence for over one year), 5 were remarkably improved (occasional recurrence within one year), 9 were improved, and 5 were inef-

fective. The total effective rate was 95.8%. The research also revealed that this therapy was not satisfying for patients suffering from pain of the whole head or occipital head and for those with a duration of disease over 5 years.

(3) Wang Didao reported 220 cases of headache treated with bleeding therapy. A blood vessel near the helix in the posterior surface of the auricle, Shenmen (MA−TF1) and Subcortex (MA−AT1) were selected. Temple (MA−AT) was added for pain of the lateral head, Occiput (MA−AT) for pain of the occipital head, Vertex (MA) and Liver (MA−SC5) for pain of the forehead, Heart (MA−IC) for patients with insomnia, and Endocrine (MA−IC3) for female patients. Method for bleeding the vessel: firstly knead the posterior surface of the auricle to make it congestive and sterilize the selected vessel, then cut the vessel quickly with a surgical blade to bleed about 30 drops followed by pressing the wound with dry cotton ball. Each of the selected auricular points was bleeded 1−2 drops. The treatment was given once every 7 days and 3 sessions constituted 1 therapeutic course. Results: 148 cases were cured, 23 were remarkably improved, 59 were improved, and 3 cases were not improved. The total effective rate was 98.6%. Follow-up on 80 cured patients confirmed that therapeutic effects were maintained in 72 patients.

15. Trigeminal neuralgia

Trigeminal neuralgia refers to recurrent and transient severe pain in the supplied area of the trigeminal nerve. It may begin at any age but is most common in middle and later life. It affects women more frequently than men. This disease is classified as primary type and secondary type. The etiology of the former is still uncertain. Possible causes include compression of blood vessels, local inflammation, viral infection, oxygen deficit and allergic reaction. The latter is often secondary to tumor, inflammation or vascular disease, which develop in the surrounding area of the trigeminal nerve, such as syringobulbia, multiple sclerosis, cerebellopontile tumor, trigeminal ganglioma, angioma, arachnoiditis and superior orbital fissure syndrome.

Among the three branches of the trigeminal nerve, the maxillary and the mandibular branches are often affected simultaneously, the maxillary branch or mandibular branch alone next, and then the maxillary, the mandibular and the ophthalmic branch simultaneously. Rarely single ophthalmic or maxillary branch is affected, and even more rarely the bilateral sides are involved simultaneously.

Essentials of diagnosis

(1) People aged over 40 years are most frequently affected. A few patients recover spontaneously.

(2) Clinical manifestations are characterized by momentary episodes of sudden tearing, lancinating, stabbing or burning facial pain that commonly arises near one side of the mouth and then shoots toward the ear, eye, or nostril on that side. Each attack lasts from several seconds to several minutes with a variable period of remission in which there is no any discomfort. A severe pain may be accompanied with reflex twitch of the facial muscles, lacrimation and conjunctival congestion.

(3) Attacks are often triggered or precipitated by touching, chewing, talking, brushing the teeth or washing the face. In order to lessen the likelihood of triggering further attacks, many patients try to hold the face still while talking.

(4) On objective examination, no positive signs can be found in the primary trigeminal neuralgia while abnormal signs in the distribution of the trigeminal nerve, such as retardation or disappearance of the corneal reflex, may be found in the secondary one.

Treatment

(1) Prescription (Fig. 4—15):

Main points: Cheek (MA—L), Jaw (MA—L), Occiput (MA—AT), Shenmen (MA—TF1), Subcortex (MA—AT1).

Supplementary points: External Nose (MA—T1), External Ear (MA—T), Central Rim (MA—AT).

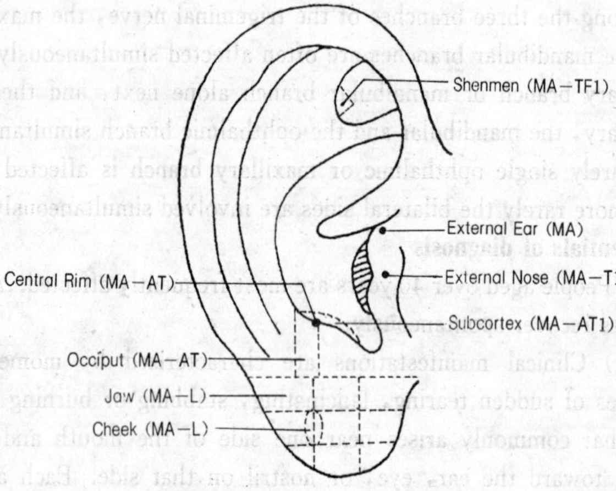

Fig. 4-15

(2) Methods:

Needling with filiform needle: In each treatment 2-3 of the main points and 1-2 of the supplementary points are selected and punctured bilaterally. Needles are retained for 30-45 minutes and manipulated with a strong stimulation technique every 5-10 minutes. The treatment can be performed once daily and 5 treatments constitute 1 therapeutic course with an interval of 5 days between courses. To improve analgesic effectiveness, It is recommended to combine auricular electroacupuncture with this therapy.

Intradermal-needle-embedding: In each treatment 2-4 of the main points and 1-2 of the supplementary points are selected and embedded with intradermal needle on the diseased side or bilateral. The needles are retained for 3-4 days and the patients are asked to press them 3-5 times daily. Five treatments constitute 1 therapeutic course with an interval of 10 days between courses.

Seed-pressing: It is better to press magnetic pellet. In each treatment all of the main points and 2-3 of the supplementary points are treated unilateral with alternating the bilateral points. The stuck pellets are changed once every 3-5 days and 10 treatments constitute 1 therapeutic course with an interval of 2-3 days between courses.

Remarks

Trigeminal neuralgia is rather intractable, body acupuncture is therefore often combined to improve therapeutic effects.

Clinical reports

Yan Shanyu reported that blockade at Trigeminal Nerve Point (MA) with lidocaine hydrochloride was effective for trigeminal neuralgia. Trigeminal Nerve Point (MA) is a sensitive point located between Central Rim (MA－AT) and Apex of Antitragus (MA－AT). Method: after sterilization, inject 0.1 ml of lidocaine hydrochlor into subcutaneous tissue of this point unilaterally or bilaterally. Treatment was performed once every 1－2 days and 5 treatments constituted 1 therapeutic course. Results: of the 12 cases treated, 7 were cured (no relapse during the follow-up period of 6 months to 2 years), 3 were improved (relapse was present within 6 months, but the frequency of attacks and severity of pain were reduced), and 2 were ineffective.

16. Sciatica

Sciatica is a common clinical syndrome, manifested by a radiating pain in the distributive region of the sciatic nerve. It can be differentiated as the primary type and the secondary type according to pathological factors, or as the root type and the trunk type according to the affected part of the nerve. Although the causes and degrees of impairment are different, pain of the lower back and leg is the common symptom. Sciatica can be caused by a variety of factors. For example, the primary sciatica may result from inflammation of the tooth, nasal sinuses or tonsil gland, which spreads to the epineurium and leads to interstitial inflammation of the sciatica nerve. In this condition, it is often accompanied with myositis or myofibrosis and aggravated by exposure to cold and dampness. There are even more causes for secondary sciatica, e.g., compression of the sciatic nerve due to diseases of the surrounding tissues, stimuli of pathological changes, or general diseases like diabetes and gout. The mechanism of sciatica is still contravertible. At present, three doctrines are proposed: physical pressure, chemical radiculoneuritis and immunoreaction.

Essentials of diagnosis

(1) Burning or lancinating pain radiates from the lower back or buttocks to the sole along the posterior side of the thigh and posterior or lateral side of the shank. The onset of root sciatica is either acute or chronic while the trunk sciatica mostly acute.

(2) Root sciatica can be aggravated by bending, cough, sneeze, etc.

(3) Lasegue's sign and Bragard's sign are positive. Root sciatica has more obvious tenderness on the diseased side of the spinal column while trunk sciatica has more obvious tenderness on the passage of the sciatic nerve.

(4) Primary diseases can be found in patients with secondary sciatica.

Treatment

(1) Prescription (Fig. 4—16):

Main points: Sciatic Nerve (MA — AH6), Shenmen (MA — TF1).

Supplementary points: Lumborsacral Vertebrae (MA — AH), Buttocks (MA — AH5), Pancreas and Gallbladder (MA — SC6), Bladder (MA—SC8).

(2) Methods:

Needling with filiform needle: Sciatic Nerve (MA — AH6) is punctured firstly. After detecting the Sciatic Nerve (MA—AH6) on the diseased side to ascertain the most painful spot, the doctor punctures it with a filiform needle. The needle is manipulated with a forceful rotating method and efforts are made to elicit a Channel transmission. Commonly, the pain will be obviously relieved following needling. If the above management fails to produce effect, Sciatic Nerve (MA — AH5) on the other side can be punctured in the same way. If there is still no response, the rest points can be punctured at last. The treatment is given once daily and 5 sessions constitute 1 therapeutic course. To promote analgesic efficacy, auricular electroacupuncture can be combined with this therapy.

Seed-pressing: It is advised to press Sciatic Nerve (MA−AH6) firstly. If the patient has no response to this treatment, the rest points can be pressed secondarily. After detecting the most sensitive point in the locus of Sciatic Nerve (MA−AH5), a vaccaria seed is stuck on the spot with plaster and pressed with strong stimulation methods to produce a hot or painful sensation in the point. The rest points are pressed with the same pressing approach. Generally, in each treatment unilateral points are treated once every 3−4 days with alternate use of the two ears, If pain is severe, bilateral points should be treated simultaneously and the seeds are renewed once every 3−5 days with an interval of two days between two successive treatments.

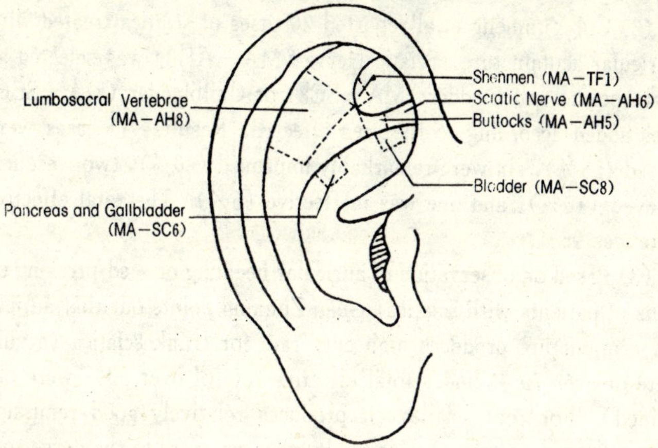

Fig. 4−16

Remarks

(1) Auricular acupuncture is effective for the treatment sciatica of both the primary type and the secondary type. For the primary type, however, the underlying disease should be treated simultaneously, otherwise satisfactory therapeutic effects will be hardly achieved or maintained.

(2) Strong stimulation to the selected point is necessary.

(3) Ascertaining the most painful spot in the locus of Sciatic

Nerve (MA—AH5) for pressing is essential for improving therapeutic effects.

Clinical reports

(1) Huang Hanxiang reported treatment of sciatica by auricular needling at bilateral Buttocks (MA—AH5), Sciatic Nerve (MA—AH6), Shenmen (MA—TF1), Knee (MA—AH3) and Ankle (MA—AH2). Shenmen (MA—TF1) was punctured horizontally to 0.7—0.8 Cun towards Gallbladder (MA—SC6) and the rest points were punctured to 0.5 Cun. The treatment was given once daily and ten treatments constituted one therapeutic course with an interval of 3—5 days between two successive courses. A total effective rate of 98% was obtained. Generally, response of the patient was present after 2—3 courses of treatment.

(2) Cui Yunmeng et al reported 20 cases of sciatica treated with auricular acupuncture. Sciatic Nerve (MA—AH6) was selected as main point, and Bladder (MA—SC8) or Gallbladder (MA—SC6) was added according to the area affected. Results: 11 cases were cured (55%), six were remarkably improved (30%), two were improved (10%), and one was ineffective (5%). The total effective rate was 95%.

(3) Based on observation of auricular needling or seed-pressing on tens of patients with sciatica, Guan Zunxing points out that auricular acupuncture produces high cure rate for trunk sciatica (a cure rate of over 70 % and a total effective rate of over 90% were obtained). For root sciatica, it produces relatively good remission rate, and cure can be obtained only when pressure to the nerve root has been removed.

17. Neurasthenia

Neurasthenia is a common kind of functional nervous diseases, mainly manifested by listlessness, lassitude, low efficiency in work, headache, insomnia, etc., but without organic changes. It is mostly found in young adults, resulting from spiritual attack, overstrain of brain and long-term mental stress, etc., which break the balance of the excito-inhibitory function of the cerebral cortex.

Essentials of diagnosis

(1) Higher excitation. It is manifested by dizziness, insomnia, dream- disturbed sleep, aversion to light and sound, blurred vision, oppression of the chest, poor self-control and symptoms of hyperactivity of the vegetative nerve such as palpitation, hectic fever of the skin or chilly hand and foot, indigestion, abdominal distention, frequent micturation, seminal emission, impotence, and irregular menstruation.

(2) Higher asthenia. The patient is not only easy to get excited but also to get tired. Other symptoms include lack of concentration, poor memory, inadequate endurance and fatigue. On examination, tendon reflex is active in the beginning but diminishes gradually along with successive percussion.

(3) Emotional disturbance. It is manifested by a tendency to get depressed, irritability and restlessness.

(4) Slow onset and long duration. The disease may last several years or even several decades with fluctuated accompanying symptoms.

(5) On examination, no manifestation of an organic disease is found.

Treatment

(1) Prescription (Fig. 4-17):

Main points: Shenmen (MA-TF1), Heart (MA-IC), Subcortex (MA-AT1), Central Rim (MA-AT), Ear Center (MA-H1).

Supplementary points: Sympathetic (MA-AH7), Ear Apex (MA-AH6), Liver (MA-SC5), Spleen (MA-IC), Kidney (MA-SC), Occiput (MA-AT).

(2) Methods:

Seed-pressing: All of the main points are selected and supplementary points are added according to TCM Syndrome Differentiation. For example, Spleen (MA-IC) is added for Deficiency of the Heart and Spleen, Kidney (MA-SC) for incoordination between the Heart and the Kidney, and Liver (MA-SC5) for depression of the Liver Qi. Magnetic pellet is the best choice for pressing of points.

In each treatment points are pressed unilaterally with alternate use of the two ears. Stuck seeds are retained for 3—5 days and the patients are asked to press them 3—5 times daily. Ten treatment constitute 1 therapeutic course with an interval of 5—7 days between courses. Since the neurasthenia patient is often pain-sensitive, seed-pressing therapy can be taken as the first choice for auricular treatment.

Drug-injection: Drugs commonly used are 0.5%—2% procaine, *Huang Qi Zhu She Ye* (Radix Astragalus Injection) and vitamin B_{12} injection. Two to three main points and 1—2 supplementary points are selected by TCM Syndrome Differentiation and 0.05—0.2 ml of drug solution is injected into each of them. Unilateral points are used in each treatment, alternating between the two ears. The treatment can be given once every 2—4 days and 7 sessions constitute 1 therapeutic course with an interval of 5 days between courses.

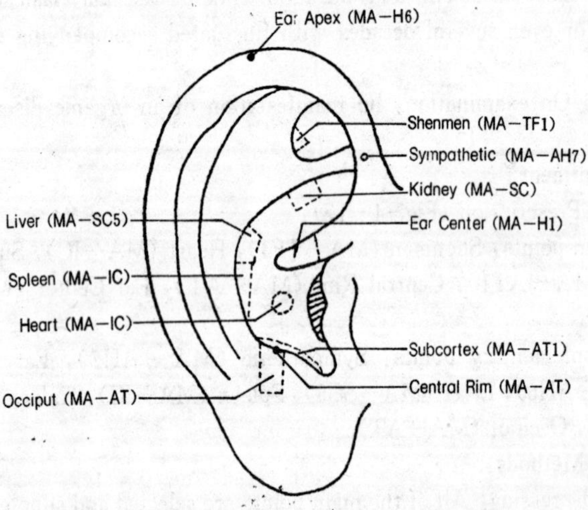

Fig. 4—17

Intradermal-needle-embedding: Two to three of the main points and 1—2 of the supplementary points are selected by TCM Syndrome Differentiation and embedded with intradermal needles. In each treatment the unilateral points are usually treated, alternating between the two ears. The needles are changed once every 3—4 days and the patients are asked to press them 3—5 times daily. Ten treatments constitute 1 therapeutic course with an interval of 7—10 days between courses.

Bleeding therapy: Two to three of the main points and 1—2 of the supplementary points are selected by Syndrome Differentiation. After routine sterilization, the practioner pricks the points with a three-edged needle or cuts them with a small surgical blade to cause bleeding. After bleeding, the wound is pressed with sterilized dry cotton ball. Beeding bleed vessels of the auricle may also be used. Method: choose a small blood vessel at the upper one-third portion of the posterior surface of the auricle; after sterilization, cut it with a surgical blade and bleed out for 2—3 ml, which can be less for weak persons and more for strong persons, and then cover it with sterilized gauge to stop bleeding. Bleeding therapy can be given once every 10—15 days and 4 treatments constitute 1 therapeutic course.

Remarks

(1) Being less pain, auricular seed-pressing therapy is easily accepted by neurasthenia patients.

(2) As a multisystem illness, neurasthenia has various and tidal symptoms and signs. Therefore, to improve therapeutic effects, TCM Syndrome Differentiation should be considered in selection of points.

(3) Ask the patients to keep away all factors unfavorable to neurasthenia.

Clinical reports

(1) Huang Lichun et al reported 166 cases of neurasthenia treated with auricular seed-pressing therapy. Main points selected were: Ear Apex (MA—AH6), Shenmen (MA—TF1), Heart (MA—IC), Occiput (Ma—AT), Subcortex (MA—AT1) and Ear Center (MA—AH1). Supplementary points were added according to TCM Syndrome Differentiation: Spleen and Small Intestine (MA—SC2) for deficiency of the Heart and the Spleen; Liver (MA—SC5) and Kidney (MA—SC) for incoordination between the Heart and the Kidney; Liver (MA—SC5) and Gallbladder (MA—SC6) for Deficiency

of the Heart Qi and the Gallbladder Qi; Liver (MA—SC5) and Sanjiao (MA—IC4) for depression of the Liver Qi; Internal Genitals (MA—TF), Endocrine (MA—IC3) and Kidney (MA—SC) for deficiency of the Kidney Yang; Stomach (MA—IC), Sanjiao (MA—IC4) and Spleen (MA—IC) for dysfunction of the Stomach Qi. In each treatment unilateral points were treated, alternating between the two ears. The stuck seeds were changed once every 3—5 days and 6 treatments constituted 1 therapeutic course. Patients received successive 1—3 courses of treatment. Results: 60 cases were clinically cured (36. 1%), 39 cases were remarkably improved (23. 5%), 43 cases were improved (25. 9%), and 24 cases were not improved (14. 5%). The total effective rate was 85. 5%.

(2) Liu Hancheng reported 105 cases of neurasthenia treated with auricular seed-pressing therapy. Main points selected were: Heart (MA—IC), Central Rim (MA—AT), Subcortex (MA—AT1), Sympathetic (MA—AH7), Root of Vagus (MA—PS) and Ear Center (MA—H1). Supplementary points were added on the basis of TCM Syndrome Differentiation: Kidney (MA—SC) and Small Intestine (MA—SC2) for hyperactivity of the Heart Yang; Liver (MA—SC5), Ear Apex (MA—H6) and Endocrine (MA—IC3) for deficiency of the Heart and Spleen; Liver (MA—SC5), Kidney (MA—SC) and Internal Genitals (MA—TF). Vaccaria seeds were used for treatment and the patients were asked to press them 4—5 times daily to produce a local sensation of soreness, numbness, distention, pain or hot. In each treatment unilateral points were treated, alternating between the two ears. The treatment was given once every other day and 10—15 treatments constituted 1 therapeutic course. Results: 64 cases were cured, 24 cases were remarkably improved, 10 cases were improved, and 7 cases were ineffective. The total effective rate was 93.35%.

(3) Gao Zhenzi reported 150 cases of neurasthenia treated with auricular seed-pressing therapy. Points selected were Shenmen (MA—TF1), Heart (MA—IC), Spleen (MA—IC), Kidney (MA—SC) and Subcortex (MA—AT1), supplemented with Lung (MA—IC1), Stomach (MA—IC), Small Intestine (MA—SC2), Occiput (MA—

AT) and Forehead (Ma—AT). Vaccaria seeds were used for treatment and the patients were asked to press them 6—8 times daily with each time lasting 5—8 minutes to produce a local hot or pain sensation. Unilateral points were pressed in each treatment, alternating between the two ears. The stuck seeds were changed once daily and 10—15 treatments constituted one therapeutic course. Results: 106 cases were remarkably improved, marked by approximate disappearance of symptoms after 1 week treatment and sleep time being increased to 6—8 hours every night; 34 cases were improved, marked by obvious improvement of symptoms and sleep time being increased to 5 hours every night; and 8 cases were not improved. The total effective rate was 94.7%.

18. Insomnia

Insomnia refers to difficulty in falling into sleep and inadequate sleep time. In mild cases, the patients feel difficult in falling into sleep, suffer from frequent alternation of sleep and wake, or only have shallow sleep or insufficient sleep time; in severe cases, the patients only have 2—3 hours' sleep each night, even no sleep for the while night. The time of sleep varies with different persons. On normal condition, children need 12—14 hours' sleep each night, young adults 7—9 hours, and elderly people 5—6 hours.

Insomnia can lie in various factors. There may be psychic or emotional factors, e.g., overstrain, worries, fright, excitement, etc.; comatic factors, e.g., pain, palpitation, cough, abdominal distention, etc.; physiological factors, e.g., noise, temperature, light, etc.; medicinal factors, e.g., administration of ephedrine and aminophyline, etc.; and pathological factors, e.g., cerebral arteriosclerosis, endocrine disorder, dysbolism, etc.

Essentials of diagnosis

(1) Shortened sleep time.

(2) Low-qualified sleep, e.g., difficulty to fall into sleep, too much dream and frequent waking-up.

(3) Accompanying symptoms include dizziness, low spirit, tiredness, lack of concentration, etc.

Treatment

(1) Prescription (Fig. 4—18):

Main points: Heart (MA—IC), Kidney (MA—SC), Shenmen (MA—TF1), Subcortex (MA—AT1), Central Rim (MA—AT).

Supplementary points: Spleen (MA—IC), Liver (MA—SC5), Pancreas and Gallbladder (MA—SC6), Stomach (MA—IC), Sanjiao (MA—IC4), Ear Apex (MA—H6), Endocrine (MA—IC3). The supplementary points are added according to TCM Syndrome Differentiation.

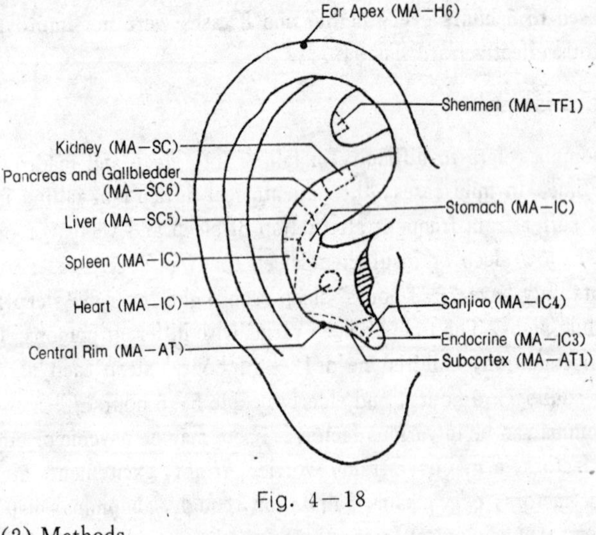

Fig. 4—18

(2) Methods:

Seed-pressing: In each treatment all of the main points and 1—2 of the supplementary points are selected. Among various kinds of auricular seeds, magnetic pellet is the best choice. Treatment is usually performed on unilateral points with alternate use of the two auricles. The stuck seeds are changed once every 3—5 days and 10 treatments constitute 1 therapeutic course. During seed retention, ask the patients to press the stuck seeds 3—5 minutes before sleep every night.

Intradermal-needle-embedding: Two to three of the main points and 1—2 of the supplementary points are selected according to Syndrome Differentiation. Intradermal needle is embedded in the selected with alternate use of the two ears. The needles are changed once every 3—4 days and 7 treatments constitute 1 therapeutic course with an interval of 5—7 days between courses. During treatment, ask the patients to press the needles 3—5 minutes before sleep every night.

Drug-injection: Drugs commonly used are 0.5%—2% procaine, *Huang Qi Zhu She Ye* (Radix Astragalus Injection) and vitamin B_{12} injection. In each treatment 2—3 of the main points and 1—2 of the supplementary points are selected according to Syndrome Differentiation, each point is injected 0.1—0.3 ml of solution. The treatment is usually performed at bilateral points once every other day. A course of treatment consists of 7 sessions with an interval of 5—7 days between courses.

Remarks

(1) Auricular acupuncture proved to be quite effective for insomnia, and in most cases obvious response will present following 2—3 treatments. If therapeutic effect is not satisfying, it should be considered whether the points, the location and/or the treatment method are proper.

(2) Since insomnia is caused by a great many factors, etiologic treatment must be given to stabilize therapeutic effects and prevent recurrence.

Clinical reports

(1) Wang Qi reported 48 cases of insomnia treated with auricular seed-pressing therapy. Points selected were Shenmen (MA—TF1), Heart (MA—IC) and Kidney (MA—SC). In each treatment two of the above three points were treated unilaterally by sticking magnetic pellets (500 GS and 3 mm in diameter), alternating between the two auricles. The seeds were changed once weekly and 1 course lasted 1 month. Results: 47 cases restored to normal sleep, and 1 case discontinued the treatment because of adverse reactions of dizziness, vomiting, perspiration, pale complexion, etc. after treatment was given.

(2) Xiao Binxiu reported 91 cases of insomnia treated with auricular intradermal-needle-embedding therapy. Points selected were Heart (MA—IC), Kidney (MA—SC), Shenmen (MA—TF1), Occiput (MA—AT) and Subcortex (MA—AT1). Intradermal needles were embedded in the above points unilaterally and they were changed every 5—7 days with alternate use of the two auricles. Seven treatments constituted one therapeutic course. After 3 successive courses of treatment, 67 cases were cured, 6 cases were improved remarkably, 10 cases were improved, and 5 cases were not improved. In contrast to two control groups, one treated with administration of *Bu Xin Wan* (Reinforcing Heart Pill) for 7—10 days and the other treated with taking librium for 3—5 days, auricular intradermal-needle-embedding therapy was most effective ($P<0.01$).

(3) He Yahong reported 200 cases of insomnia treated with auricular seed-pressing therapy. Points selected were Heart (MA—IC), Kidney (MA—SC), Subcortex (MA—AT1) and Shenmen (MA—TF1). Vaccaria seeds were stuck to the above points bilaterally and they were changed once every 5 days. Ask the patients to press the stuck seeds 3 times daily with each point being pressed 30 times to produce a local sensation of hot, pain, soreness and/or numbness. Results: 120 cases were improved remarkably, 70 cases were improved, and 10 cases were not improved. The total effective rate was 95%.

(4) Zhang Xiaofen reported that auricular seed-pressing therapy is superior to Western medicine in treating insomnia. In the auricular seed-pressing treatment group (n=218), vaccaria seeds were used to press the follow points: Heart (MA—IC), Shenmen (MA—TF1), Occiput (MA—AT), Forehead (MA—AT), Central Rim (MA—AT) and Subcortex (MA—AT1) as main points, and Kidney (MA—SC), Liver (MA—SC5), Spleen (MA—IC) and Stomach (MA—IC) as supplementary points. Results: 136 cases were cured (62.4%), 76 cases were improved (34.8%), and 6 cases were not improved (2.8%). The total effective rate was 97.2%. In the Western medicine treatment group (n=60), administration of diazepamum (valium) 5—15 mg or 10% chloral hydrate 10—30 ml

once per night. Results: 10 cases were cured (16.7%), 10 cases were improved (16.7%), and 40 cases were not improved (66%). The therapeutic effects in the two groups was significantly different in favor of the auricular seed-pressing therapy.

19. Periarthritis of shoulder

Periarthritis of shoulder refers to the chronic inflammation of the soft tissues around the shoulder, e.g., muscle, tendon and synovium, clinically characterized as pain and dysfunction of the shoulder joint. Seen mostly in those aged over 50 years, it is considered to be a chronic degenerative condition induced or aggravated by overstrain, trauma, exposure to cold, etc.

Essentials of diagnosis

(1) It occurs in the middle or elder age, developing gradually or induced by overstrain, trauma, exposure to cold, etc.

(2) Pain of the shoulder joint, which, in severe condition, may radiate to the neck, forearm and hand. The pain turns to the better in the day time and worse at night.

(3) Limited movement of the shoulder joint. In the initial stage, dysfunction of the shoulder joint may not be clear. After repeated attacks, the movement of the shoulder joint will be limited obviously, and the patient may even feel difficult to comb his hair, to wash his face and to brush his teeth.

(4) Muscular atrophy may be seen in patients with a long duration of the disease.

(5) Physical examination finds extensive tenderness around the shoulder joint.

Treatment

(1) Prescription (Fig. 4-19):

Main points: Shoulder (MA-SF4), Shenmen (MA-TF1), Adrenal Gland (MA-T).

Supplementary points: Subcortex (MA-AT1), Kidney (MA-SC), Liver (MA-SC5), Ear Apex (MA-H6), Endocrine (MA-IC3).

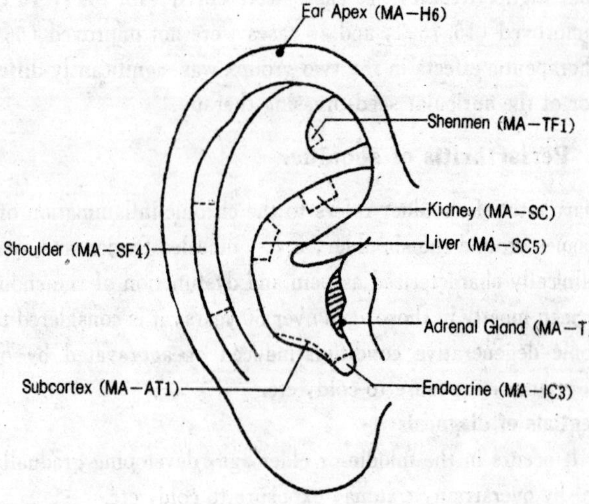

Fig. 4-19

(2) Methods:

Needling with filiform needle: In each treatment all of the main points and 2—3 of the supplementary points are selected according to TCM Syndrome Differentiation, alternating between the two ears. After detecting the sensitive spot in the point locus and applying routine sterilization, points are punctured with filiform needles. Except Kidney (MA—SC), all other points are stimulated with a strong manipulation technique. While manipulating the needles ask the patients to move the affected shoulder joint positively. The needles are retained for 20—30 minutes. The treatment can be performed once daily and 5—10 treatments constitute 1 therapeutic course.

Electroacupuncture: Two to three of the main points and 1—2 of the supplementary points are selected in each treatment. After needles are inserted into the selected points, one of the main points and one of the supplementary points are connect to an electric stimulator for electric stimulation. The dense wave and dense-disperse wave are applied alternately to stimulate the points for 30 minutes. During retention of the needles, ask the patient to move the affected shoulder joint as far as possible. The treatment can be given once daily and ten times constitute one therapeutic course. Auricular electroacupuncture has rather good analgesic efficacy. It is therefore suitable for patients with obvious pain. After the pain is relieved, auricular seed-pressing therapy can be used as a substitute.

Seed-pressing: All of the main points and 2—3 of the supplementary points are selected according to TCM Syndrome Differentiation. After sensitive spots in the point loci are detected, vaccaria seed or magnetic pellet is stuck to them. Points are treated on one side points in each treatment, alternating between the bilateral points. The stuck seeds are changed once every 3—5 days and the patients are asked to press the stuck seeds 3—5 times daily. While performing pressing, the patients should be advised to do movement of the affected shoulder joint as far as possible.

Remarks

(1) Most patients of the first attack can be cured completely by auricular acupuncture. For those with repeated attacks and obvious limitation of the shoulder joint, more exercise of the affected joint is essential for restoration of the joint function.

(2) Auricular acupuncture is very effective for relieving pain, but not satisfying for improving limitation of the joint movement.

Clinical reports

(1) It is reported that auricular reflection therapy has favorable effect on stage I periarthritis of shoulder. Points selected were Clavicle (MA—SF5), Shoulder (MA—SF4), Shenmen (MA—TF1), etc. Electric stimulation was applied to the selected points in combination with topical application of pepper ointment and massage. All of the 56 patients with periarthritis of shoulder were cured after 3—6 treatments, marked by complete pain relief and restoration of movement of the shoulder joint. The total effective rate was 100%. Follow-up of 6 months revealed that except two patients who had relapse, the therapeutic effects were maintained in all other patients.

(2) Chen Shouji reported 50 cases of periarthritis of shoulder treated with auricular electroacupuncture. Points selected were

Shoulder (MA－SF4), Clavicle (MA－SF5), Subcortex (MA－AT1) and Shenmen (MA－TF1). Results: 30 cases were cured, 14 cases were improved remarkably, 4 cases were improved, and 2 cases were ineffective. The effectiveness was superior to that of a control group ($P<0.005$). Patients in the control group was treated with CO_2 laser radiation at the following points: Yunmen (LU 2), Jianyu (LI 15), Quyuan (SJ 13), Tianzong (SJ 11) and Jianzhen (SJ 9).

20. Irregular menstruation

Irregular menstruation refers to the abnormality of menstrual cycle, quantity, color and quality, accompanied with other symptoms. Temporary irregular menstruation resulting from alternation of climate, environment, emotion, etc. is not considered as illness. Irregular menstruation mentioned here mainly concerns with abnormal cycle of menses, including preceded menstrual cycle, delayed menstrual cycle and indefinite menstrual cycle. It is caused by an imbalance between hypothalamus, pituitary and ovary. External environment, psychic and emotional state, physical condition and other endocrine glands can affect the function of the above organs and subsequently bring about irregular menstruation.

Essentials of diagnosis

(1) Preceded menstrual cycle. Menstruation is advanced by 7 days or even 10 days, often accompanied with fresh-red or purple color of the blood.

(2) Delayed menstrual cycle. Menstruation is delayed by over 7 days, or even occurs once every 40－50 days, often accompanied with light or dark red color of the blood.

(3) Indefinite menstrual cycle. Menstruation is advanced sometimes and delayed sometimes by over 7 days, often accompanied with either massive or scanty volume and either dark or light red color of the blood.

Treatment

(1) Prescription (Fig. 4－20):

Main points: Internal Genitals (MA－TF), Endocrine (MA－

IC3), Liver (MA−SC5), Spleen (MA−IC).

Supplementary points: Kidney (MA−SC), Central Rim (MA−AT), Sympathesis (MA−AH7), Subcortex (MA−AT1).

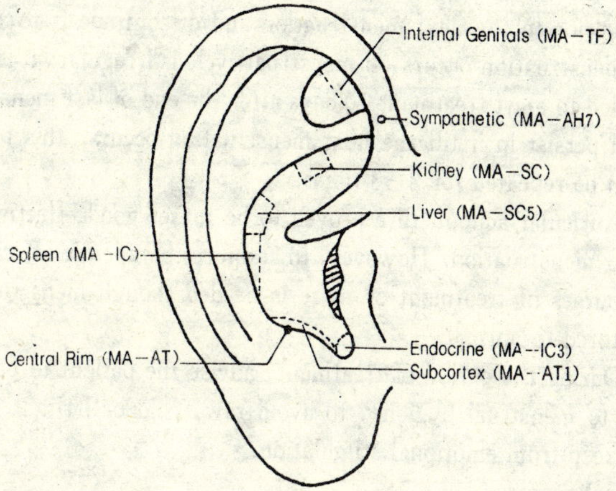

Fig. 4−20

(2) Methods:

Needling with filiform needle: In each treatment 2−3 of the main points and 1−2 of the supplementary points are selected unilaterally according to Syndrome Differentiation with alternate use of the two auricles. When performing treatment, it is advised to detect the sensitive spot in the point locus first and then puncture it with filiform needle after routine sterilization. The needles are retained for 20−30 minutes and treatment is performed once daily with 1 course consisting of 10 sessions. It is better to start the treatment 10 days after menstruation and continue it until the next menstruation occurs. This procedure of treatment can be repeated for 2−3 times.

Seed-pressing: In each treatment all of the main points and 2−3 of the supplementary points are selected according to Syndrome Differentiation with alternate use of the two auricles. After the sensitive spots in the point locus are detected, vaccaria seeds are stuck to them and they are changed once every 2−3 days with 10 times as 1 therapeutic course. During retention of the seeds, the patients are asked to press the stuck points 3—5 times daily. The treatment can be repeated for 2—3 courses.

Remarks

(1) If menstrual cycle is regular, it is advised to start treatment 10 days prior to the next menstruation and discontinue it to 1 day before menstruation occurs. If menstrual cycle is irregular, it is recommended to start treatment 10 days after the end of last menstruation and persist in it till the next menstruation occurs. this procedure can be repeated for 2—3 times.

(2) Auricular acupuncture proved to be rather good effective for irregular menstruation. However, to stabilize therapeutic effects, 1—2 courses of treatment or more is needed though menstruation has restored to normal.

(3) During the period of treatment, advise the patient to pay attention to menstrual hygiene, to avoid raw, cold or irritant food, and to keep from emotional stimulation.

Clinical reports

(1) Zhen Ji reported 77 cases of irregular menstruation treated by pressing vaccaria seeds at auricular points. Points selected were: Shenmen (MA—TF1), Liver (MA—SC5) and Kidney (MA—SC) as main points, and Subcortex (MA—AT1) or Endocrine (MA—IC3) as supplementary point. Treatment was performed at the above points unilaterally with alternate use of the two auricles. However, if menstruation did not occur on the expected date, treatment was given at the bilateral points, and bilateral points were also treated simultaneously for preceded menstruation. During the period of treatment, the patients were required to press the stuck seeds 3—5 times daily with each time lasting 5 minutes. After 3—6 courses of treatment, 25 cases were improved remarkably, 49 cases were improved, and 3 cases were not improved.

(2) Hou Jianxiong reported 36 cases of irregular menstruation treated with auricular needling. Points were selected according to TCM Syndrome Differentiation: Sanjiao (MA—IC4), Groove of Posterior Surface (MA—PS), Homeostasis Point (MA), Liver (MA—SC5) and Liver Yang 1—3 for Blood-Heat type of preceded

menstruation; Heart (MA－IC), Spleen (MA－IC), Kidney (MA－SC), Hormone Point (MA) and Endocrine (MA－IC3) for type of Blood Deficiency; Internal Genitals (MA－TF), Hormone Point (MA), Adrenal Gland (MA－T), Pituitary Gland (MA), Ovary (MA), Kidney (MA－SC) and Spleen (MA－IC) for type of Deficiency Cold due to insufficiency of Qi and Blood in patients suffering from delayed menstruation; Thyroid Gland (MA), Adrenal Gland (MA－T), Pituitary Gland (MA), Thalamus (MA), Angle of Superior concha (MA－TF), Sanjiao (MA－IC4), Ovary (MA), Lung (MA－IC1) and Spleen (MA－IC) for type of Phlegm-Dampness; Liver (MA－SC5), Sanjiao (MA－IC4), Endocrine (MA－IC3), Ovary (MA), Kidney (MA－SC) and Spleen (MA－IC) for type of Liver Qi depression in patients suffering from indefinite menstruation; and Adrenal Gland (MA－T), Angle of Superior concha (MA－TF), Thyroid Gland (MA), Hormone Point (MA), Kidney (MA－SC) and Spleen (MA－IC) for type of Kidney Deficiency. Results: 5 cases were improved remarkably, 25 cases were improved, and three cases were ineffective.

21. Dysmenorrhea

Dysmenorrhea refers to severe pain in the lower abdomen and lumbosacral region prior to, or during menstrual period, which affects the patient's daily life and routine work. It is classified into two types: primary and secondary. The primary type, also called functional dysmenorrhea, refers to those without obvious pathological changes of the pelvic organs. The secondary type refers to those caused by organic pathological changes of the genital organs, e.g., endometriosis, pelvic inflammation and submucosal myoma of the uterus. Dysmenorrhea discussed here mainly refers to the primary type.

Essentials of diagnosis

(1) Most patients develop this disease in the first 2 years after menarche.

(2) Paroxysmal and spasmodic pain appears in the lower abdomen 1－2 days or several hours prior to onset of menstruation and may

radiate to the lumbosacral region, vulva, anus and even medial aspect of the thigh and lower abdomen. The pain usually lasts for 2—3 days.

(3) It may be accompanied with vomiting, nausea, diarrhea or constipation, and even collapse in severe case.

(4) No distinct organic focus is found by gynecological examination.

Treatment

(1) Prescription (Fig. 4—21):

Main points: Internal Genitals (MA—TF), Endocrine (MA—IC3), Central Rim (MA—AT), Shenmen (MA—TF1), Angle of Superior Concha (MA—TF).

Supplementary points: Sympathetic (MA—AH7), Liver (MA—SC5), Kidney (MA—SC), Subcortex (MA—AT1).

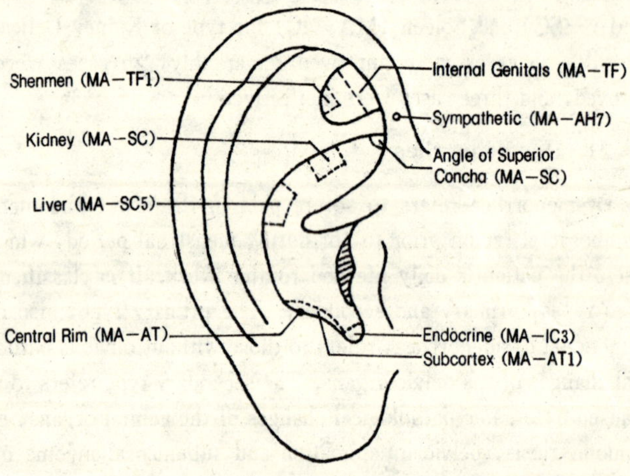

Fig. 4—21

(2) Methods:

Needling with filiform needle: In each treatment 2—3 of the main points and 1—2 of the supplementary points are selected bilaterally according to Syndrome Differentiation. After detecting the sensitive spot in the point locus and applying routine sterilization, the doctor punctures the points with filiform needle. The needles are retained for 30—45 minutes. The treatment can be performed once daily. It is advised to start the treatment 3—5 days prior to the next menstrual cycle and continue it until the end of the menstruation.

Intradermal-needle-embedding: Two to three of the main points and 1—2 of the supplementary points are selected, alternating between the bilateral points. After detecting the sensitive spots in the point locus, intradermal needle is embedded in them. In each treatment unilateral points are treated for mild cases with alternate use of the two auricles while bilateral points are treated for severe cases. The needles are retained for 3—5 days and the patients are asked to press them 3—5 times daily. It is recommended to start the treatment 5 days before the expected date of the next menstruation and continue it until the end of the menstruation.

Seed-pressing: In each treatment all of the main points and 2—3 of the supplementary points according to Syndrome Differentiation, alternating between the bilateral points. After sensitive spots of the point locus are detected, vaccaria seeds are stuck to them and they are changed once every 2—3 days. Ask the patients to press the stuck points 3—5 times daily. For patients with severe pain, the bilateral points should be treated simultaneously.

Remarks

(1) Auricular acupuncture proved to be quite effective for dysmenorrhea. However, attention should be paid to the treatment opportunity in order to improve therapeutic effects. The treatment procedure is advised to be repeated for 2—3 times regardless of whether pain is relieved.

(2) It is necessary to explain to the patients that the syndrome is a physiological phenomenon of menstruation, which helpful to relieve their tension occurring prior to and during menstrual period and improve therapeutic effects.

Clinical reports

(1) Zhong Yuanming et al reported 50 cases of dysmenorrhea treated with auricular seed-pressing therapy. Points selected were Endocrine (MA—C3), Internal Genitals (MA—TF), Shenmen (MA—TF1), Kidney (MA—SC) and Liver (MA—SC5). Vaccaria

seeds were stuck to the above bilateral points and each point was pressed for 0. 5—1 minutes. If pain was not relieved, press those points 10—15 times for each at intervals of 5—10 minutes. Seeds were retained for 12—24 hours. After 1—4 treatments, 49 cases recovered and only 1 case failed to respond. The total effective rate was 98%.

(2) Liu Qingshan et al reported 30 cases of primary dysmenorrhea treated with auricular needling. Internal Genitals (MA—TF) was selected as main point, supplemented with Endocrine (MA—IC3), Subcortex (MA—AT1) and Sympathetic (MA—AH7). The above points were punctured with filiform needles. The needels were retained for 15 — 30 minutes and were manipulated with rotating method. One therapeutic course consisted of 3—5 days. Results: 25 cases were improved remarkably and 9 cases were improved.

(3) Liu Shizhong reported 100 cases of dysmenorrhea treated auricular seed-pressing therapy. Points were selected according to TCM Syndrome Differentiation. For accumulation of Cold and Dampness, Internal Genitals (MA—TF), Endocrine (MA—IC3), Central Rim (MA — AT) and Ovary (MA) were used as main points, supplemented with Sympathetic (MA—AH7) and Shenmen (MA — TF1); for stagnation of Qi and Blood, Internal Genitals (MA—TF), Sympathetic (MA—AH7), Central Rim (MA—AT) and Ovary (MA) were used as main points, supplemented with Spleen (MA—IC) and Liver (Ma—SC5); and for Deficiency of Qi and Blood, Internal Genitals (MA—TF), Kidney (MA—SC), Liver (MA — SC5) and Endocrine (MA — IC3) were used as main points, supplemented with Sympathetic (MA—AH7) and Shenmen (MA—TF1). Vaccaria seeds used to press the selected points and the stuck seeds were changed once every 3 days. The above points were treated unilaterally in each treatment, alternating between the 2 auricles. Ask the patients to press the stuck seeds 3—5 times daily. If the patient was in the acute stage of attack, bilateral points were treated simultaneously and the stuck seeds were changed once every other days. One course of treatment consisted of 10 treatments with an interval of 3—5 days between 2 successive courses.

Results: 817 cases were cured (81.7%), 159 cases were improved remarkably (15.9%), 20 cases were improved (2.0%), and 4 cases were ineffective (0.5%). The total effective rate was 99.6%.

22. Amenorrhea

Amenorrhea is a common symptom, defined as a condition that a female aged over 18 years (in some countries, such as the USA, the age is stipulated as 16 years) has not established menstruation, or that the menstruation once established have ceased for more than three months. The former is called primary amenorrhea while the latter secondary amenorrhea. However, those present in the period of pregnancy, lactation and menopause must be ruled out, which are considered a physiological phenomenon. Amenorrhea can be caused by a variety of factors, and in fact all disorders of the uterus, ovary, pituitary, thalamus and cerebral cortex can yield amenorrhea. Amenorrhea resulting from blockage of the genital tract due to congenital defect or acquired injury of the certain part of the lower genital tract such as hymen, vagina and cervix is called pseudo-amenorrhea, which is excluded in this discussion.

Essentials of diagnosis

(1) Case history is of importance. For primary amenorrhea, a detailed knowledge about growth, developmental process, including intelligence, nutrition and spiritual state, healthy condition in childhood and whether being attacked by serious diseases, is very important. For secondary amenorrhea, the patient should be inquired about menarche, menstrual condition before occurrence of amenorrhea, duration of amenorrhea, whether there have been induction factors like spiritual stimulation and alteration of living environment, and whether the patient has experienced abortion, uterine curettage, difficult labor, postpartum hemorrhage or infection.

(2) On examination, attention should be paid to the general development, nutritional state, intelligent condition and whether there is secretion of milk, etc.

(3) Measurement of hormones of the pituitary gland and ovary is helpful to ascertain the causes of amenorrhea.

Treatment

(1) Prescription (Fig. 4—22):

Main points: Internal Genitals (MA—TF), Endocrine (MA—IC3), Central Rim (MA—AT), Kidney (MA—SC).

Supplementary points: Liver (MA—SC5), Spleen (MA—IC), Subcortex (MA—SC).

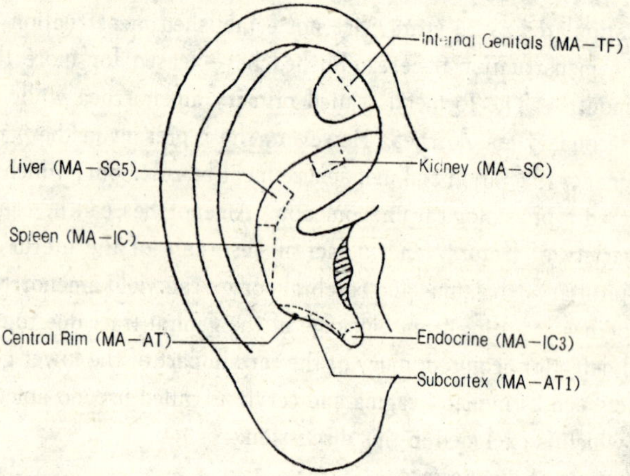

Fig. 4—22

(2) Methods:

Needling with filiform needle: All of the main points and 1—2 of the supplementary points are selected according to Syndrome Differentiation. After routine sterilization, the practioner punctures the selected points with filiform needle which is retained for 20—30 minutes. Commonly, one auricle is treated in each treatment, alternating between the two auricles. The treatment can be performed once daily or every other day and 10 sessions constitute 1 course with an interval of 5—7 days between courses.

Intradermal-needle-embedding: Two to three of the main points and 1—2 of the supplementary points are selected according to Syndrome Differentiation. After routine sterilization, intradermal needles are embedded in the selected points and they are changed once every 3—5 days. One auricle is used in each treatment, alternating between the two auricles. Five sessions constitute 1 therapeutic course with an interval of 10 days between courses.

Seed-pressing: All of the main points and 1—2 of the supplementary points are selected according to Syndrome Differentiation. Alternating between the bilateral points, points are pressed with vaccaria seeds and the stuck seeds are changed once every 3—5 days. Ten treatments constitute 1 therapeutic course. During the period of seed retention, ask the patients to press the points 3—5 times daily.

Remarks

(1) Auricular acupuncture proved to be effective for secondary amenorrhea. In order to stabilize therapeutic effects, it is necessary to continue the treatment for 2—3 courses after menstruation has restored.

(2) The patients are advised to keep a smooth and light wood and keep from overstrain and unfavorable emotional stimulation.

Clinical reports

(1) Zhao Guang reported 40 cases of irregular menstruation and amenorrhea treated with auricular seed-pressing therapy. Main points selected were Uterus (MA), Ovary (MA) and Endocrine (MA—IC3), supplemented with Liver (MA—SC5), Kidney (MA—SC) and Heart (MA—IC). Stick vaccaria seeds on the above points unilaterally with alternate use of the bilateral points. Change the stuck seeds once every 3 days with 10 treatments constituting 1 therapeutic course. Results: 38 cases were improved, marked by reappearance of menstruation; and the remaining 2 cases were not improved.

(2) Tian Conghe reported that auricular needling is quite effective for amenorrhea. Points used were Uterus (MA), Central Rim (MA—AT), Ovary (MA), Endocrine (MA—IC3) and Kidney (MA—SC). Two to three of the above points were selected in each treatment and punctured with filiform needles. Retain the needles for 30 minutes and manipulate them with rotating method 2—3 times during retention period. Treatment was given once daily and 10—12 treatments constituted 1 therapeutic course. The author pointed out that auricular needling was suitable for functional amenorrhea but

not satisfying for severe secondary amenorrhea.

23. Dysfunctional uterine bleeding

Dysfunctional uterine bleeding refers to abnormal bleeding of the uterus resulting from regulatory disorder of the endocrine system but without any distinct organic pathological changes of the internal and external genitals. It is characterized by indefinite menstrual cycle, delayed menstrual period and irregular uterine bleeding. Dysfunctional uterine bleeding is divided as an ovulatory type and a non-ovulatory type. The ovulatory type is mostly seen in women of child-bearing period, caused by dysfunctional corpus luteum or prolonged atrophy of corpus luteum; the non-ovulatory type is commonly encountered in women of adolescence and climacterium, resulting from premature regulatory function between hypothalamus and pituitary gland in adolescence, or atrophy of ovary in climacterium.

Essentials of diagnosis

(1) Non-ovulatory type: It is marked by disorder of menstrual cycle, indefinite menstrual period and massive or scanty bleeding. Some patients show constant bleeding after a temporary loss of menstruation from several weeks to several months, and some have increased quantity of bleeding and prolonged menstrual period but normal menstrual cycle. Gynecological examination finds no specific abnormality. Basal body temperature demonstrates monophasic type, smear of vaginal exfoliated cells finds non-ovulatory periodic change, and premenstrual cervical mucus shows fernlike crystal or non-typical.

(2) Ovulatory type: It comprises two conditions: dysfunctional corpus luteum and incomplete atrophy of corpus luteum. The former is marked by shortened menstrual period, difficulty in conception, and susceptibility of abortion. There is no distinct abnormality found on gynecological examination. Basal body temperature displays by phasic curve, but the temperature goes up slowly and the amplitude is insufficient. Uterine curettage done in menstrual period or within 6 hours after onset of menstruation shows inadequate sec-

retary reaction of the endometrium. The latter is marked by prolonged menstrual period and massive quantity of bleeding. Basal body temperature displays by phasic curve, but the uterine curettage done on the 5th or 6th day after menstruation displays that secretary reaction of the endometrium still exists.

Treatment

(1) Prescription (Fig. 4—23):

Main points: Internal Genitals (MA—TF), Endocrine (MA—IC3), Adrenal Gland (MA—T), Central Rim (MA—AT).

Supplementary points: Liver (MA—SC5), Spleen (MA—IC), Kidney (MA—SC).

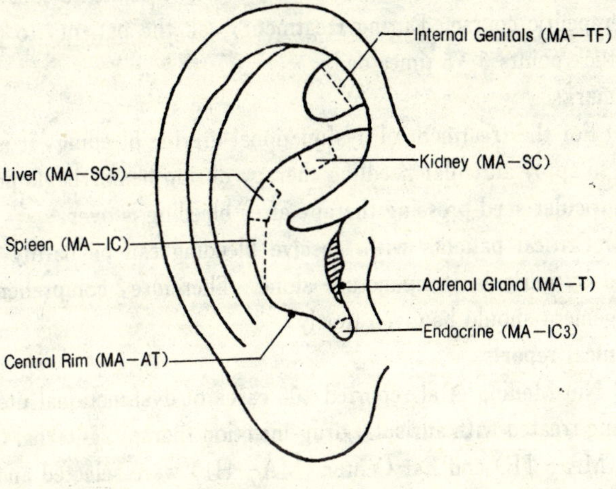

Fig. 4—23

(2) Methods:

Needling with filiform needle: All of the main points and 1—2 of the supplementary points are selected according to Syndrome Differentiation. One auricle is used in each treatment, alternaing between the two auricles. After routine sterilization, the selected points are punctured with filiform needle, which is retained for 20—30 minutes. For manipulation of the needle, strong stimulation methods are applied for Excess type while week for Deficiency type. The treatment can be performed once daily and 10 sessions constitute 1 course.

Drug-injection: Vitamin K_3 solution is commonly used. In each treatment 2—3 of the main points and 1—2 of the supplementary points are selected unilaterally according to Syndrome Differentiation, with alternate use of the bilateral points. Drug solution is injected into the selected points with 0.3 ml for each point. The treatment can be given once daily and 10 sessions constitute 1 course.

Seed-pressing: In each treatment all of the main points and 1—2 of the supplementary points are selected unilaterally according to Syndrome Differentiation, alternating between the two auricles. The selected points are pressed with vaccaria seeds and the stuck seeds are renewed once every 3—5 days. Ten treatments constitute 1 therapeutic course. During treatment, ask the patients to press the stuck points 3—5 times daily.

Remarks

(1) For the treatment of dysfunctional uterine bleeding, it is advised to apply auricular needling therapy during hemorrhagic period and auricular seed-pressing therapy after bleeding is over.

(2) Critical patients with massive bleeding can be hardly controlled by auricular acupuncture alone. Therefore, comprehensive management should be given timely.

Clinical reports

(1) Niu Meiling et al reported 100 cases of dysfunctional uterine bleeding treated with auricular drug-injection therapy. Internal Genitals (MA—TF) and Ear Center (MA—H1) were selected and injected 0.1 ml of vitamin K_3 solution for each point. Treatment was given once daily for successive three sessions. Results: 68 cases were cured, 17 case were improved remarkably, and 4 cases were ineffective. The total effective rate was 96%.

(2) Yang Lanxu reported 82 cases of dysfunctional uterine bleeding treated with auricular seed-pressing therapy. Main points used were Spleen (MA—IC), Subcortex (MA—AT1), Kidney (MA—SC) and Heart (MA—IC). Supplementary points were added according to Syndrome Differentiation: Stomach (MA—IC) and Pancreas and Gallbladder (MA—SC6) for disorder of the Stomach Qi,

and Shenmen (MA－TF1) and Central Rim (MA－AT) for insomnia. Results: 36 cases were cured (43.9%), 18 improved remarkabl'y (20.9%), 16 improved (19.4%), and 12 not improved. The total effective rate was 85.3%.

24. Premenstrual syndrome

Premenstrual syndrome refers to a series of repeated symptoms and signs appearing during the 7－10 days before the onset of menses and subsiding when menstruation occurs, such as tension, lack of concentration, irritability, depression, headache, dizziness, insomnia, distending pain in breast, and even abdominal distention, vomiting and general edema. For a few patients, those symptoms may develop at other time of menstrual cycle. With unclear causes, premenstrual syndrome is mostly found in women aged between 30－45 years. The majority of the patients have normal menstruation and have no relation with marriage and pregnancy.

Essentials of diagnosis

(1) Nervous and psychic symptoms, e.g., a tendency to excitement, anger, fright and worry, lassitude, and lethargy. Diffuse headache is common and migraine is occasional.

(2) Symptoms of retention of water and sodium, mostly seen as subcutaneous edema of the lower limbs, and edema of the eyelids, hands and feet the second. The patients may get weight gain for 1－3 kg owing to edema, and the edema will subdue gradually after onset of menstruation.

(3) Distending pain or tenderness of the breast, distention of the lower abdomen, heavy sensation in the pelvic cavity, soreness of the lumbar region, vomiting, nausea, etc.

(4) Painful joints.

(5) A few patients may develop urticaria, fever, acne, ulcerative stomatitis, etc.

(6) Symptoms is recurrent along with menstrual cycle.

Treatment

(1) Prescription (Fig. 4－24):

Main points: Endocrine (MA－IC3), Shenmen (MA－TF1),

Sympathetic (MA—AH7), Subcortex (MA—AT1).

Supplementary points: Internal Genitals (MA—TF), Heart (MA—IC), Liver (MA—SC5), Spleen (MA—IC), Kidney (MA—SC).

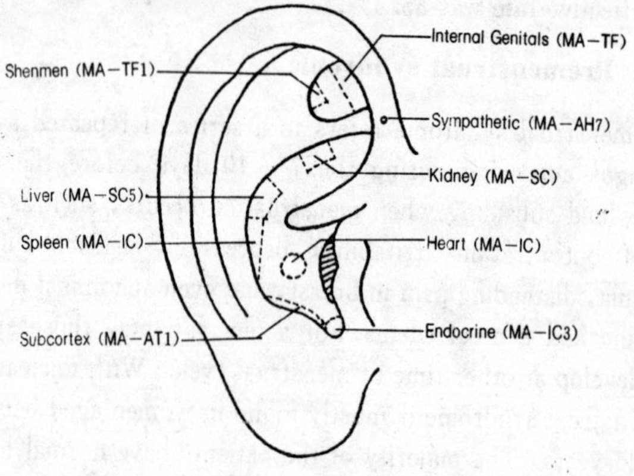

Fig. 4—24

(2) Methods:

Needling with filiform needle: According to TCM Syndrome Differentiation, 2—3 of the main points and 1—2 of the supplementary points are selected unilaterally in each treatment with alternate use of the bilateral points. After routine sterilization, the selected points are punctured with filiform needle, which is retained for 20—30 minutes. The treatment can be performed once daily with 10 sessions as 1 course of treatment. Bilateral points can also be treated simultaneously with the treatment given once every other day.

Seed-pressing: All of the main points and 1—2 of the supplementary points are selected according to Syndrome Differentiation and pressed with vaccaria seed or magnetic pellet. Generally, unilateral points are treated in each treatment with alternate use of the bilateral pointsand, the stuck seeds are changed once every 3—5 days. Ten treatments constitute 1 therapeutic course. During treatment, ask the patients to press stuck points 3—5 times daily.

Remarks

(1) More attention should be paid to the treatment of opportunity. It is recommended to start treatment 7—10 days prior to the ex-

pected date of the next menstruation and persist in the treatment till the menstruation occurs. This procedure can be repeated for 2—3 times.

(2) Careful evaluation of the patient, with understanding, explanation, and reassurance is of first importance.

(3) Advise the patient to keep a daily diary of all symptoms for 2—3 months, to help in evaluating the timing and characteristics of the symptoms. Psychotherapy may be helpful for some women or couples.

(4) It is helpful for the patients to relieve their symptoms if they reduce intaking of water (500 ml is proper per day) and salt.

Clinical report

Guan Zunxin reported 7 cases of premenstrual syndrome treated with auricular needling. Of the 5 cases manifested mainly by psychic symptoms, 3 cases were cured and 2 improved remarkably. The rest 2 cases clinically marked by retention of water and sodium were improved remarkably.

25. Menopausal syndrome

The term "menopause" refers to the final cessation of menstruation, either a normal part of aging or as the result of surgical removal of both ovaries. In a broader sense, as the term is commonly used, it denotes a 1—3 years period during which a woman adjusts to a diminishing and then absent menstrual flow and the physiological changes that may be associated-hot flushes (feelings of intense heat over the trunk and face, with flushing of the skin and sweating), night sweats, and vaginal dryness or soreness with coitus.

The average age at menopause is between 45—55 years. A part of women smoothly tides over this period, but a part of women suffers from symptoms of sexual hormone decline and dysfunction of the vegetative nerve, which are called menopausal syndrome or syndromes of around menopause.

Essentials of diagnosis

(1) Cessation of menstruation. Menstrual cycles generally be-

come irregular as menopause approaches. Anovular cycles occur more often, with irregular cycle length and occasional menorrhagia. Menstrual flow usually diminishes in amount owing to decreased estrogen secretion, resulting in less abundant endometrial growth. Finally, cycles become longer, with missed periods or episodes of spotting only. When no bleeding has occurred for 1 year, the menopausal transition can be said to have occurred.

(2) Women aged between 45 – 66 years or have undergone ovariectomy present hot flushes, sweating, emotional instability, lack of concentration, insomnia, irritability, a crying tendency, dizziness, headache, low sexual function, etc.

(3) Atrophy of the genitals and breast found by examination.

(4) Osteoporosis and hyperlipemia.

Treatment

(1) Prescription (Fig. 4–25):

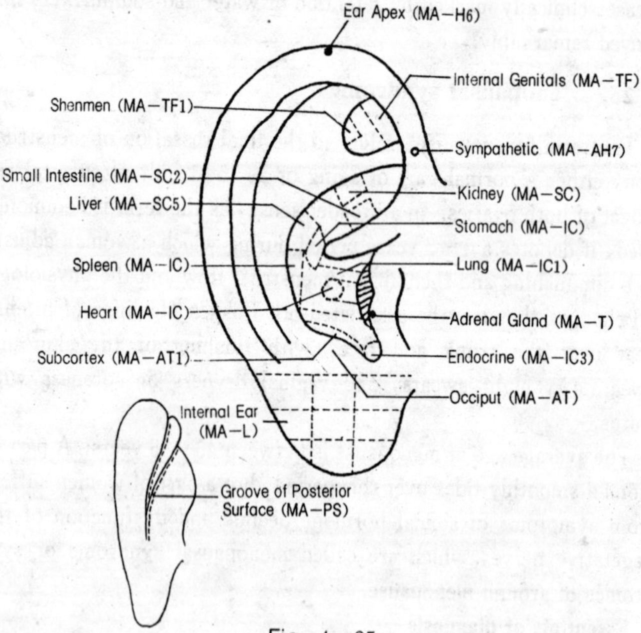

Fig. 4–25

Main points: Internal Genitals (MA－TF), Endocrine (MA－IC3), kidney (MA－SC).

Supplementary points: Heart (MA－IC), Shenmen (MA－TF1) and Subcortex (MA－AT1) for emotional instability; Heart (MA－IC), Sympathetic (Ma－AH7) and Small Intestine (MA－SC2) for palpitation; Ear Apex (MA－H6) and Groove of Posterior Surface (MA－PS) for hypertension; Liver (MA－SC5) and Spleen (MA－IC) for dysfunctional uterine bleeding; Sympathetic (Ma－AH7) and Lung (MA－IC1) for tide fever; Internal Ear (MA－L) and Adrenal Gland (MA－T) for tinnitus; and Stomach (MA－IC) and Occiput (MA－AT) for nausea and vomiting.

(2) Methods:

Seed-pressing: All of the main points are used, and the supplementary points are added according to Syndrome Differentiation. With alternate use of the bilateral points, the selected are pressed with vaccaria seed or magnetic pellet and the stuck seeds are changed once every 3－5 days. Fifteen treatments constitute 1 therapeutic course. During treatment, ask the patients to press the stuck seeds 3－5 times daily. Ear Apex (MA－H6) is usually pricked with a three-edged needle to cause bleeding.

Needling with filiform needle: All of the main points are used, and the supplementary points are added according to Syndrome Differentiation. After routine sterilization, the selected points are punctured with filiform needle, which is retained for 20－30 minutes. For manipulation of the needles, the strong stimulation methods are applied for Excess type while weak for Deficiency type. The treatment can be performed once daily with 10 sessions as 1 course of treatment. Bilateral points can also be treated simultaneously with treatment given once every other day.

Remarks

(1) Since symptoms and manifestations of menopausal syndrome are complicated, the selection of points should be adjusted with different symptoms.

(2) Explain to the patient that menopause is a physiological period in life, which is helpful to relieve the patient's emotional stress

and worries.

(3) Patients should be advised to have light food and prevent hot and spicy food.

Clinical reports

(1) Liu Jifang reported 50 cases of menopausal syndrome treated with auricular seed-pressing therapy. Main points selected were Uterus (MA), Ovary (MA), Endocrine (MA－IC3), Subcortex (MA－AT1), Shenmen (MA－TF1), Sympathetic (Ma－AH7), Kidney (NA－SC) and Occiput (MA－AT). Supplementary points were added according to Syndrome Differentiation: ① Lung (MA－IC1), Central Rim (MA－AT) and Internal Ear (MA－L) for deficiency of the Kidney Yin; ② Spleen (MA－IC) and Exciting Point (MA) for deficiency of the Kidney Yang; ③ Liver Yang1 (MA), Liver Yang2 (MA), Gallbladder (MA－SC6) and Sanjiao (MA－IC4) for depression of the Liver Qi; and ④ Liver (MA－SC6) and Eye (MA－L) for deficiency of both the Kidney Yin and Liver Yin. Vaccaria seeds were pressed onto the selected points unilaterally with alternate use of the bilateral points. The treatment was given once every other day and 14 sessions constituted 1 course with an interval of 5 days between 2 successive courses. During the treatment, the patients was required to press the stuck seeds themselves 5－7 times daily. After 2 courses of treatment, 38 cases were improved remarkably, 8 cases improved, and 4 cases not improved. The total effective rate was 92%.

(2) Gu Shenchun reported 56 cases of menopausal syndrome treated with auricular seed-pressing therapy. Main points selected were Uterus (MA), Shenmen (MA－TF1), Endocrine (MA－IC3), Subcortex (MA－AT1), supplemented with Liver (MA－SC5), Gallbladder (MA－SC6), Sanjiao (MA－IC4), Heart (MA－IC), Spleen (MA－IC), Stomach (MA－IC), Kidney (NA－SC), Large Intestine (MA－SC4) and Bladder (MA－SC8). Vaccaria seeds were used to press the above points. Results: 31 cases recovered (55.4%), 16 cases improved remarkably (28.6%), 4 cases improved (7.1%), and 5 cases failed to respond (8.8%). The total effective rate was 91.1%.

26. Hyperthyroidism

Hyperthyroidism is one of the common endocrine disorders resulting from excessive secretion of thyroid hormone due to hyperfunction of the thyroid gland. It is clinically manifested by symptoms of high metabolism, hyperactivity of the nervous system and cardiovascular function, and thyroid enlargement. The cause of the disease is various and the pathology is marked by diffuse, nodular or mixed thyroid enlargement, and pathologic changes of various organs and tissues.

Essentials of diagnosis

(1) Manifestations resulting from elevated basal metabolism, e. g., aversion to heat, profuse sweating, warm, humid and flushed skin, lower fever, palpitation, intake of excess food but with susceptibility to hunger and obvious weight loss, and fatigue.

(2) Symptoms of hyperactive sympathetic nerve, e. g., nervousness, excitement, hasty speech and action, wary, suspicion, and even depression or mania. In some cases, shaking of hands and active tendon reflex may be seen.

(3) Thyroid enlargement. About 90% of the patients has diffuse enlargement of the thyroid gland in varying degrees. About 70% of the patients can be auscultated murmur, of which half can be palpitated tremor.

(4) Symptoms of the eye, e. g., gaze or lessened nictitation, tremor of the eyelid and exophthalamus.

(5) Pretibial myxedema seen in about 2%—3% patients.

(6) Symptoms of the cardiovascular system, e. g., increased pulse pressure, tachycardia, arrhythmia and atrial fibrillation, etc.

(7) Symptoms of the digestive system, e. g., dyspepsia, diarrhea, etc.

(8) Symptoms of the reproductive system, e. g., irregular menstruation, infertility, etc.

(9) Laboratory test shows increased function of the thyroid gland in taking ^{131}I and high content of serum T_3 and T_4.

Treatment

(1) Prescription (Fig. 4—26):

Main points: Neck (MA—AH10), Endocrine (MA—IC3), Sympathetic (Ma—AH7), Subcortex (MA—AT1).

Supplementary points: Heart (MA — IC), Shenmen (MA — TF1), Spleen (MA—IC), Liver (MA—SC5), Mouth (MA—IC5), Hunger Point (MA).

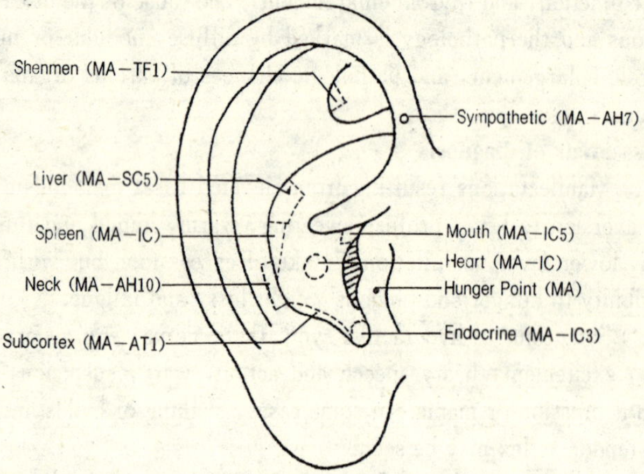

Fig. 4—26

(2) Methods:

Needling with filiform needle: According to TCM Syndrome Differentiation, in each treatment 2—3 of the main points and 1—2 of the supplementary points are selected unilaterally with alternate use of the bilateral points. After routine sterilization, the sensitive spots in the locus of the selected points are punctured with filiform needles and retain them for 20—30 minutes. The treatment can be performed once daily or every other day with 10 sessions as 1 course of treatment. Bilateral points can also be treated simultaneously if symptoms are obvious.

Seed-pressing: All of the main points and 1—2 of the supplementary points are selected according to Syndrome Differentiation and pressed with vaccaria seed or magnetic pellet. The stuck seeds are changed once every 3 — 5 days with alternate use of the bilateral points and 10 treatments constitute 1 therapeutic course. During treatment, ask the patients to press the stuck points 3—5 times daily.

Intradermal-needle-embedding: According to TCM Syndrome Differentiation, in each treatment 2—3 of the main points and 1—2 of the supplementary points are selected unilaterally with alternate use of the bilateral points. After routine sterilization, intradermal needle is embedded in the sensitive spots of the locus of the selected points. The needles are changed once every 3—5 days and 10 times constitute 1 course with an interval of 10 days between courses.

Remarks

(1) Auricular acupuncture proved effective for improving clinical symptoms of hyperthyroidism. However, a rather long course of treatment is necessary. Therefore, in clinical treatment, two groups of auricular points are often formulated and used alternately.

(2) Ask the patient to avoid emotional irritation and pay attention to diet.

27. Myopia

Myopia is a kind of ametropic ophthalmopathy, manifested as clear in seeing distant objects but obscure in seeing nearby objects. Clinically, it is classified into two type: true myopia and pseudomyopia. The former results from the condition that the optic axis is too long or the cornea is too powerful in refraction, which causes the external parallel light to be focused before they reach the retina. The latter, also called spasm of the accommodation, is due to overuse of focus adjustment as the result of reading at too close distance. Cyclospasm and the subsequent increase in convexity of lens cause the external parallel light to focalize in front of the retina. Myopia results from heredity and harmful habits of using eyes such as poor illumination, improper sitting posture, overuse of the eyes, etc.

Essentials of diagnosis

(1) In seeing objects with naked eyes, it is clear for the near but obscure for the distant. The eye is susceptible to tiredness.

(2) There is no obvious abnormality of the outward appearance of the eye, but exophthalmus may be seen in cases with high myopia.

(3) When harmful habits or overuse of eyes are removed, vision can improves for pseudomyopia but not for true myopia.

Treatment

(1) Prescription (Fig. 4—27):

Main points: Eye (MA—L1), Liver (MA—SC5), Kidney (MA—SC), Shenmen (MA—TF1).

Supplementary points: Eye1 (MA—L), Eye2 (MA—L), Sympathetic (Ma—AH7), Subcortex (MA—AT1).

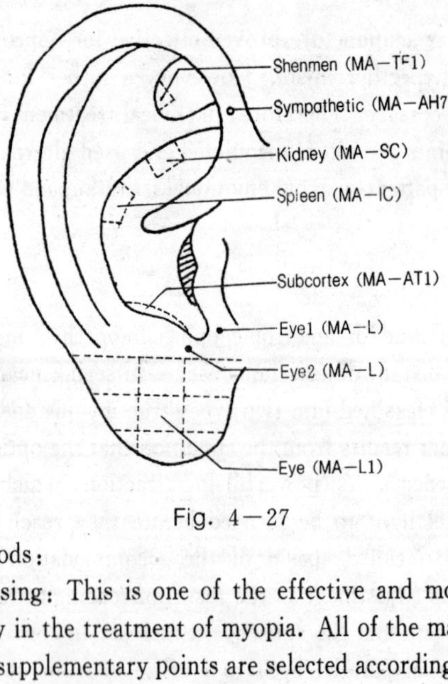

Fig. 4—27

(2) Methods:

Seed-pressing: This is one of the effective and most commonly used therapy in the treatment of myopia. All of the main points and 1—2 of the supplementary points are selected according to Syndrome Differentiation. After detecting the sensitive spots in the loci of the selected points, vaccaria seed or magnetic pellet is stuck onto them unilaterally with alternate use of the bilateral points. The seeds are changed every 3—5 days and 10 sessions constitute 1 course with an interval of 10 days between courses. During treatment, ask the patients to press the stuck seeds 3—5 times daily. When pressing the points, the patient should be advised to close his eyes and pay his though to the eyes. It is better to produce a hot sensation in the auricle and a soreness, distention or hot sensation in the eyes when pressing.

Intradermal-needle-embedding: All of the main points and 1—2 of the supplementary points are selected according to Syndrome Differentiation. After detecting the sensitive spots in the locus of the selected points and applying routine sterilization, the doctor embeds intradermal needle in them. Usually, points are treated unilaterally in each treatment, alternating between the bilateral points. The needles are changed once every 3—5 days and 5 sessions constitute 1 course.

Needling with filiform needle: All of the main points are used and punctured bilaterally in each treatment. Needles are retained for 20—30 minutes. The treatment can be performed once daily or every other day with 10 sessions as 1 course of treatment. Auricular needling is usually given in the initial period of treatment, and after therapeutic effect is obtained, it is substituted with auricular seed-pressing therapy to stabilize the efficacy.

Remarks

(1) Auricular acupuncture produces rapid effectiveness for pseudomyopia, and an obvious improvement can be obtained after only 1—2 treatments. For true myopia, satisfactory therapeutic effects are hardly achieved by single auricular acupuncture.

(2) Ask the patients to pay more attention to the proper use of eyes,

Clinical reports

(1) Liu Jing et al reported 1459 cases of juvenile myopia treated with auricular seed-pressing therapy. Main points selected were Eye (MA—L1), Eye1 (MA—L) and Eye2 (MA—L), supplemented with Occiput (MA—AT), Liver (MA—SC5) and Kidney (MA—SC). Vaccaria seeds were used to press the selected points unilaterally with alternate use of the bilateral points. Seeds were changed every 7 days and one-month treatment was taken as a therapeutic course. Patients were ask to press the stuck seeds themselves 3—5

times daily. Results of 1823 eyes: 253 eyes restored to normal (vision was elevated to over 1.0), 1319 eyes were improved (vision was elevated by over 1—2 lines in visual acuity test chart), and 493 eyes were not improved. The total effective rate was 82.45%. Clinical observation also demonstrated that the effects were satisfactory in persons aged between 7—19 years but declined if the patient was over 20 years old, indicating that the younger the patient, the better the effect.

(2) Bao Shuncai et al reported 1617 cases of juvenile myopia treated with auricular intradermal-needle-embedding therapy. Patients were classified into 5 types and treated with points selected based on Syndrome Differentiation. ① Liver type: select Liver (MA—SC5) as main point and Eye (MA—L1), Gallbladder (MA—SC6), Eye1 (MA—L) and Eye2 (MA—L) as supplementary points; ② Heart type: select Heart (MA—IC) as main point and Eye (MA—l), Small Intestine (MA—SC4), Eye1 (MA—L) and Eye2 (MA—L) as supplementary points; ③ Kidney type; select Kidney (MA—SC) as main point and Eye (MA—l), Bladder (MA—SC8), Eye1 (MA—L) and Eye2 (MA—L) as supplementary points; ④ Lung type: select Lung (MA—IC1) as main point and Eye (MA—l), Large Intestine (MA—SC4), Eye1 (MA—L) and Eye2 (MA—L) as supplemented points; and ⑤ Spleen type: select Spleen (MA—IC) as main point and Eye (MA—l), Stomach (MA—IC), Eye1 (MA—L) and Eye2 (MA—L) as supplementary. After sterilization, filiform needles were punctured into the selected points accurately, and then fixed with adhesive plaster. Points were treated unilaterally with alternate use of the bilateral points. The needles are changed once per week with six times as a therapeutic course. Results: 359 cases restored to normal (vision was elevated to over 1.0), accounting for 22.2%; 962 cases were improved, accounting for 59.49%; and 296 cases failed to respond, accounting for 18.3%. The total effective rate was 81.69%.

(3) Zhang Yanhua et al reported that therapeutic effects of auricular seed-pressing therapy in the treatment of myopia varied with different materials though they were all effective. Results revealed

that medicinal pills such as *Yi Shi Wan* (Improving Vision Pill) and *Ling Bao Wan* (Precious Pill) were more effective than plant seeds, and that alternate use of medicinal pills was much more effective than single use of one.

(4) Lai Xinping conducted a comparative study on effects of auricular seed-pressing and body needling. In the auricular seed-pressing group consisting of 236 cases (468 eyes), points selected were Eye (MA–L1), Heart (MA–IC), Liver (MA–SC5), Kidney (MA–SC), Eye1 (MA–L) and Eye2 (MA–L). Results: 98 eyes restored to normal or improved remarkably and 349 eyes improved; the total effective rate was 95%. In the body needling group consisting of 48 cases (96 eyes), points selected were Chengqi (ST 1), Cuanzhu (BL 2), Fengchi (GB 20) and Hegu (LI 4), which were alternated with Jingming (BL 1), Yifeng (SJ 17) and Guangming (GB 37). Besides, Sanyinjiao (SP 6), Zusanli (ST 36), Ganshu (BL 18) and Shenshu (BL 23) were added according to TCM Syndrome Differentiation. Results: 18 eyes restored to normal and 69 eyes improved; the total effective rate was 90.04%. There was no significant difference between effective rates of the two groups ($P < 0.05$). However, since auricular seed-pressing therapy is convenient to perform and does not produce injury, pain and infection, it is therefore more valuable to be advocated.

28. Acute conjunctivitis

Acute conjunctivitis, also called acute catarrhal conjunctivitis or popularly named *Hong Yan Bin* (Pink-Eye Disease) in China, is the most common eye disease, characterized by obvious congestion and mucopurulent secretion of the eyes. Most cases are exogenous and due to bacterial, viral, or chlamydial infection, although endogenous inflammation may occur. The mode of transmission of infectious conjunctivitis is usually direct contact via fingers, towels, handkerchiefs, etc. to the fellow eyes or to other persons. It occurs mostly in spring and autumn.

Essentials of diagnosis

(1) Chief symptoms are severe itching and foreign body and/or

burning sensation of the eyes, and even photophobia and lacrimation.

(2) Examination shows swelling of the eyelids, congestion of the conjunctiva, especially in the fornical conjunctiva, and purulent discharges presenting in the surface of the conjunctiva.

(3) Sudden onset. It usually reaches its maximum within 3－4 days and then subdues gradually, lasting for 10－14 days.

Treatment

(1) Prescription (Fig. 4－28):

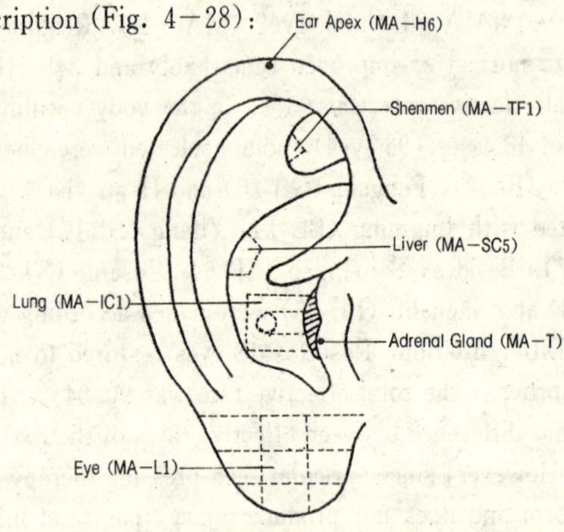

Fig. 4－28

Main points: Ear Apex (MA－H6), Eye (MA－L1).

Supplementary points: Adrenal Gland (MA－T), Liver (MA－SC5), Lung (MA－IC1), Shenmen (MA－AT1).

(2) Methods:

Bleeding therapy at auricular points: After detecting the sensitive spots in the selected points and performing routine sterilization, the doctor pricks the points with a three-edged needle to bleed 4－5 drops in each point. Ear Apex (MA－H6) can be bleeded 7－8 drops. Commonly, the treatment is applied to the unilateral points once daily and 4 sessions constitute 1 course, alternating between the bilateral points.

Bleeding therapy at veins of the posterior auricular surface: An obvious shallow vein in the upper part of the posterior auricular surface is selected. After kneading it to make it congestive and applying routine sterilization, the doctor pricks it with a three-edged needle to bleed 7—8 drops. To facilitate bleeding, the doctor can squeeze the pricked point. The treatment can be given at unilateral points once per day with alternate use of the two auricles and 4 times constitute 1 therapeutic course.

Needling with filiform needles: All of the main points and 2—3 of the supplementary points are selected according to Syndrome Differentiation. After routine sterilization, needles are inserted into the selected points and then manipulated with a strong stimulation technique. The needles are retained for 30—45 minutes. Commonly, the treatment is given at unilateral points once daily in each treatment, with alternate use of the bilateral points.

Remarks

(1) Auricular acupuncture proved remarkably effective for acute conjunctivitis and a marked improvement is often obtained after 1—2 treatments.

(2) For patients in the acute stage of attack, bleeding therapy is the best choice, while for those in the remission stage, auricular seed- pressing therapy is more suitable.

Clinical reports

(1) Hu Hongying reported 112 cases of acute conjunctivitis treated with bleeding therapy at Ear apex (MA—H6). Method: sterilize the point routinely, and then prick it with a three-edged needle to bleed 3—5 drops with the help of squeezing. After treatment, 74 cases recovered, marked by disappearance of redness, swelling, pain and photophobia of the eyes; 36 cases improved, marked by reduced symptoms; and 1 case failed to respond. The total effective rate was 99.1%.

(2) Yan Yong reported that bleeding at veins of the posterior auricular surface was effective for infectious conjunctivitis. Method: select an obvious blood vessel near the helix in the auricular posterior surface and knead it for 1—2 minutes to cause congestion, then prick it with a three-edged needle to bleed 2—3 drops. Among the 45 cases treated, 44 were cured, of which, 27 cases were cured only

with 1 treatment, 12 with 2 treatments, and 5 with 3 treatments.

(3) Yang Dongrong et al reported 30 cases of acute conjunctivitis treated with auricular needling. Main points selected were Ear Apex (MA−H6) and Eye (MA−L1), supplemented with Groove of Posterior Surface (MA−PS). Points were pricked with a three-edged needle to a depth of 0.1−0.2 cm and then squeezed to bleed several drops. Results: 13 cases were cured with 1 treatment, 12 cases with 2 treatments and 4 cases with 3 treatments, but 1 case was not improved.

29. Chronic rhinitis

Chronic rhinitis refers to chronic inflammation of the nasal mucosa and submucous layer. It is classified into two type, simple and hypertrophic. The latter often results from the former. There are three kinds of main causes. ① Local factors, e.g., repeated attack of acute rhinitis or long- term stimulation of surrounding focus; ② Occupational or surrounding factors, e.g., long-term intaking of polluted air and sudden change of temperature or humidity of environment; ③ General factors, e.g., some chronic or infectious diseases, malnutrition and long-term habits of smoking and drinking.

Essentials of diagnosis

(1) Nasal obstruction and running nose: The nasal obstruction usually turns for the better in the day time or when the patient is at working or doing exercise while turns to the worse at night or the patient is sitting quietly or exposing to cold. Hypertrophic rhinitis shows severe nasal obstruction, which is usually persistent.

(2) It may be accompanied with headache, dizziness, insomnia, hyposmia, etc.

(3) Examination of the nasal cavity shows swelling of the nasal mucosa with profuse sticky secretion.

Treatment

(1) Prescription (Fig. 4−29):

Main points: Internal Nose (MA−T), External Nose (MA−T1), Lung (MA−IC1), Adrenal Gland (MA−T).

Supplementary points: Shenmen (MA−TF1), Subcortex (MA−

AT1), Heart (MA—IC), Spleen (MA—IC), Kidney (MA—SC), Occiput (MA—AT), Forehead (MA—AT).

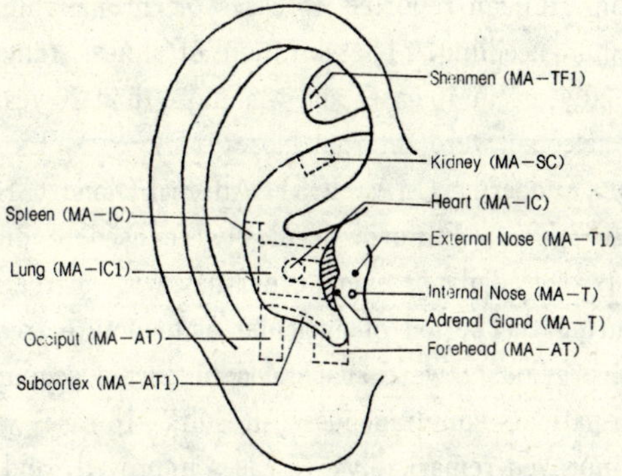

Fig. 4—29

(2) Methods:

Seed-pressing: All of the main points and 2—3 of the supplementary points are selected according to Syndrome Differentiation. After cleaning the auricle with alcohol cotton ball, the doctor sticks vaccaria seed or magnetic pellet on the selected points unilaterally, alternating between the bilateral points. The seeds are changed once every 3—5 days and 10 sessions constitute 1 course. Ask patients to press the stuck seeds themselves 3—5 times daily during the period of treatment.

Needling with filiform needles: According to Syndrome differentiation, 2—3 of the main points and 1—2 of the supplementary points are selected for each treatment. With alternate use of the bilateral points, treatment is given once daily and 10 sessions constitute 1 course. If bilateral points are treated simultaneously, it is advised to give the treatment once every other day or alternate two groups of points.

Remarks

(1) Although auricular acupuncture produces therapeutic effects quickly in improving symptoms of chronic rhinitis, 2—3 treatment courses or more are necessary to stabilize the therapeutic effective-

ness.

(2) Adrenal Gland (MA−T) is not proper for atrophic rhinitis.

Clinical reports

(1) Wang Huijuan reported 45 cases of chronic rhinitis treated with auricular needling. The duration of illness ranged from 5 months to 20 years in 40 cases and was more than 20 years in 5 cases. Points selected were Internal Nose (MA−T), External Nose (MA−T1), Endocrine (MA−IC3), Adrenal Gland (MA−T) and Lung (MA − IC1). Filiform needles were used to puncture the above points once daily or every other day with 5 treatments as a course. During the period of auricular acupuncture treatment, all drugs used previously were suspended but scalp acupuncture was given in 15 patients simultaneously. Results: 16 cases were cured, ten cases improved remarkably, 15 cases improved, and four cases not improved.

(2) Liu Zhuming reported 196 cases of chronic rhinitis treated with auricular seed-pressing therapy. Points selected were Internal Nose (MA−T), External Nose (MA−T1), Lung (MA−IC1), Adrenal Gland (MA−T) and Forehead (MA−AT). Treatment was applied to the bilateral points and the seeds were changed once every 5 days. Four sessions constitute 1 therapeutic course with an interval of 2−4 days between 2 courses. Ask the patients to press the stuck seeds at lest 3 times daily. Results: 12 cases were cured (6.1%), marked by disappearance of symptoms, complete recovery of the nasal function and no relapse within 6 months; 121 cases were improved (61.7%), marked by disappearance of symptoms and basical recovery of the nasal function; 61 cases were improved (31.1%), marked by disappearance of subjective symptoms and partial recovery of the nasal function; and 2 cases were ineffective. The total effective rate was 99%.

30. Allergic rhinitis

Allergic rhinitis results from allergic reaction due to dust, pollen, food or bacteria. It is characterized by sudden onset and withdrawal of sneeze, accompanied with profuse watery discharge. During remission period there is no obvious signs while in attack stage there are pallor and edema of the nasal mucosa, increased number of eosinophils in the nasal secretions. Allergic rhinitis can occur all the year round or in a certain season, and affect people at any age but more frequent in juvenile.

Essentials of diagnosis

(1) Itching of the nose, sneeze and watery discharge. Prior to attack, itching of the nose is presents, followed by sudden onset of successive sneeze and watery discharge. Because the discharge lacks mucoitin, the towel stained with nasal discharge will not become hard after it is dry.

(2) Nasal obstruction. Being varying in severity, it may be intermittent or persistent and affect nostril either unilaterally or bilaterally.

(3) Hyposmia or anosmia.

(4) It may be accompanied with headache, tinnitus, lacrimation, chronic cough, etc.

(5) Nasal examination shows swelling of the nasal mucosa with purplish red or grey color.

Treatment

(1) Prescription (Fig. 4—30):

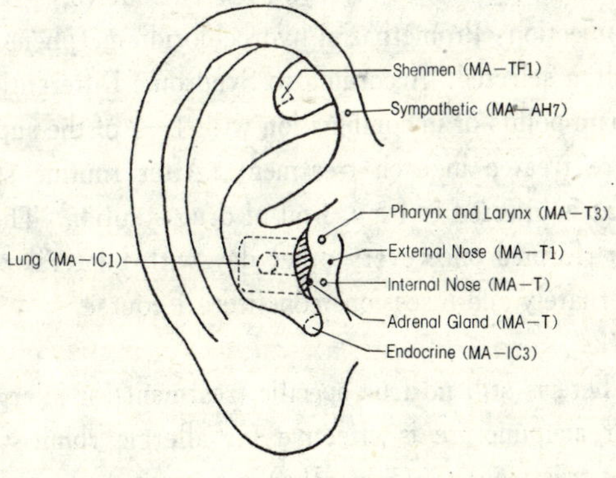

Fig. 4—30

Main points: Internal Nose (MA—T), External Nose (MA—

T1), Lung (MA－IC1) and Adrenal Gland (MA－T).

Supplementary points: Endocrine (MA－IC3), Sympathetic (MA－AH7), Shenmen (MA－TF1), Pharynx and Larynx (MA－T3).

(2) Methods:

Seed-pressing: All of the main points and 2－3 of the supplementary points are selected according Syndrome Differentiation. Magnetic pellet is the best choice but vaccaria seed is applicable. With alternate use of the bilateral points, treatment is given once every 3－5 days and 10 sessions constitute 1 therapeutic course with an interval of 10 days between 2 courses. If attacks are frequent, the bilateral points should be treated simultaneously and the stuck seeds are changed once every 3 days with an interval of 1 day between 2 successive treatments. During treatment, ask the patient to press the stuck seeds 3－5 times daily.

Needling with filiform needle: According to Syndrome Differentiation, 2－3 of the main points and 1－2 of the supplementary points are selected for each treatment. After routine sterilization, the selected points are punctured with filiform needles, which are retained for 20－30 minutes. The treatment is given once daily with alternate use of the bilateral points, or once every other day if bilateral points are treated simultaneously. Ten treatments constitute 1 therapeutic course with an interval of 10 days between courses.

Drug-injection: Promethazini hydrochloridium (phenergan) injection is often selected. According to Syndrome Differentiation, 2－3 of the main points or in combination with 1－2 of the supplementary points are treated in each treatment. After routine sterilization, each point is injected 0.1－0.3 ml of drug solution. The treatment can be performed once every other day with bilateral points being used alternately and 6 sessions constitute 1 course.

Remarks

(1) There is still no true specific treatment for allergic rhinitis. Auricular acupuncture is effective for allergic rhinitis, however, persistent treatment (3－6 months) is necessary.

(2) For seasonal rhinitis, it is advised to start treatment 3－6 months before the beginning of the season.

Clinical reports

(1) Qiao Yuzhen reported 100 cases of rhinitis treated with auricular seed-pressing therapy. Main points selected were Internal Nose (MA—T), Trachea (MA—IC2) and Lung (MA—IC1). Supplementary points were added on the basis of accompanying symptoms. Central Rim (MA—AT) and Subcortex (MA—AT1) were added for headache; Temple (MA—AT), Cheek (MA—L), Occiput (MA—AT) and/or Vertex (MA) were added according to the area of headache; Apex of Antitragus (MA—AT) and Shenmen (MA—TF1) were added for cough and asthma; and Large Intestine (MA—SC4) and Rectum (MA—H2) were added for constipation. With alternate use of the bilateral points, vaccaria seeds were stuck to the selected points and they were changed once every 3 days with 6 sessions as a course. Ask the patients to press the stuck seeds 3—5 times daily during treatment. Results of the 100 cases: 85 cases were improved remarkably (complete disappearance of symptoms), 10 improved, and 5 failed to respond. Most of the patients noticed disappearance of watery discharge following two treatments.

(2) Qin Zhao et al reported 21 cases of allergic rhinitis treated with auricular seed-pressing therapy. Main points selected were Wind Stream (MA—SF), Lung (MA—IC1), Internal Nose (MA—T) and External Nose (MA—T1), supplemented with kidney (MA—SC), Spleen (MA—IC), Adrenal Gland (MA—T) and Subcortex (MA—AT1). Vaccaria seeds were used for treatment and 5—6 of the above points were treated unilaterally in each session. Seeds were changed once every 3 days with 6 sessions as a course. Ask the patients to press the stuck seeds 3—5 times daily during the period of treatment. Results of 21 cases: 8 cases improved remarkably, 12 improved and 1 failed to respond. The total effective rate was 95.2%. Provocative test of the nasal mucosa was significant difference before and after treatment ($0.01 < P < 0.02$). In contrast with a control group ($n=22$) treated with nasal drip of 0.01% ketotifen solution, the efficacy of the auricular seed-pressing therapy was superior to that of the drug ($P < 0.05$).

(3) Peng Lihua reported 337 cases of allergic rhinitis treated with

auricular seed-pressing therapy. Main points selected were Lung (MA—IC1), Trachea (MA—IC2), Shoulder (MA—SF4), Fingers (MA—SF1), Internal Nose (MA—T), External Nose (MA—T1). Supplementary points were added according to Syndrome Differentiation: Spleen (MA—IC), Stomach (MA—IC) and Sanjiao (MA—IC4) for deficiency of the Spleen and Stomach, and Liver (MA—SC5), Kidney (MA—SC), Sympathetic (MA—AH7) and Shenmen (MA—TF1) for interior Heat resulting from Yin insufficiency. Vaccaria seeds were stuck to the selected points with *She Xiang Zhuang Gu Dao* (Plaster for Strengthening Bones Mainly with Moschus). Results of the 337 cases: 161 case were cured (44.8%), 130 improved remarkably (38.6%), 45 improved (13.3%), and 11 not improved. The total effective rate was 96.7%. In random 50 subjects, measurement of IgA, IgG and IgM, which were lower previously in the majority of subjects, restored to normal after treatment. Analysis of the values revealed a significant difference before and after treatment of auricular seed-pressing ($P<0.01$).

31. Tinnitus and deafness

Tinnitus and deafness are two most common symptoms in diseases of the ear. Tinnitus refers to a sound perception in the ear or the head though no corresponding sound source in the external environment; and deafness refers to hypoacusis, which is also popularly called *Zhong Ting* (Decline of Hearing) for mild cases and *Er Long* (Deafness) for severe cases in TCM. Though tinnitus and deafness are different, frequently they exists simultaneously.

Tinnitus can be classified as vibrational tinnitus and non-vibrational tinnitus. The former results from a sound from the internal ear or surrounding organs while the latter from disorders of the cochlear spiral organ, internal tympatic muscles, tympatic plexus, etc. Tinnitus may be objective (heard by the examiner) or subjective. Objective tinnitus is uncommon and is usually caused by transmitted vascular vibrations in the blood vessels of the head and neck or by rhythmic rapid contractions of the muscles of the soft palate or middle ear. The examiner can often hear the sound through a stethoscope placed over the ear or can see movement of the eardrum or palate. Subjective tinnitus usually accompanies hearing loss or other disease of the external, middle, or inner ear. It is a common symptom in middle-aged or elderly adults. Although the cause is unknown, tinnitus is presumed to be due to irritation of nerve endings in the cochlea by degenerative vascular or vasomotor disease.

Deafness is divided into two type: conductive and sensory. The conductive deafness may be congenital, due to malformations of the external or middle ear. Trauma may produce perforation of the eardrum or disruption of the ossicular chain. Inflammatory middle ear disease may produce serious otitis media, acute or chronic purulent otitis media, or adhesive otitis media. The sensory deafness may also be congenital, due to birth trauma, maternal rubella, etc.; or it may be due to traumatic injury to the inner ear or eighth nerve, vascular disorder with hemorrhage or thrombosis in the inner ear, ototoxic drugs and other chemical agents, etc.

Treatment

(1) Prescription (Fig. 4−31):

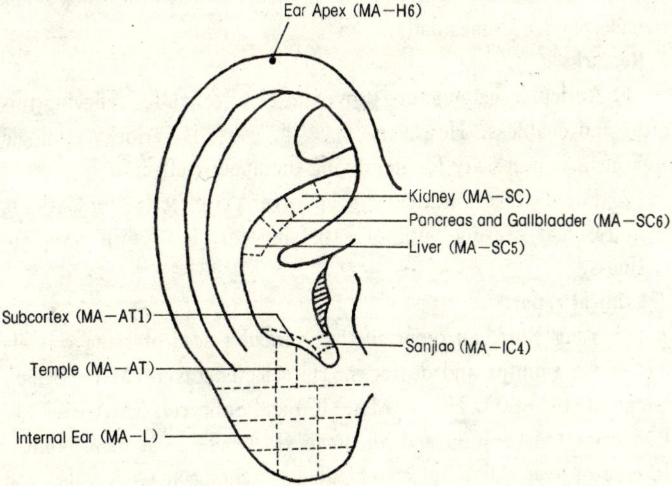

Fig. 4−31

Main points: Internal Ear (MA−L), Liver (MA−SC5), Kidney

(MA—SC), Subcortex (MA—AH1).

Supplementary points: Ear Apex (MA—H6), Temple (MA—AT), Sanjiao (MA—IC4), Pancreas and Gallbladder (MA—SC6).

(2) Methods:

Seed-pressing: All of the main points are used and 2—3 of the supplementary points are selected according Syndrome Differentiation. Magnetic pellet is the best choice, and vaccaria seed is applicable if magnetic pellet is not available. With alternate use of the bilateral points, the treatment is given once every 3—5 days and 10 treatments constitute 1 therapeutic course at an interval of 7 days between courses. During treatment, ask the patients to press the stuck seeds themselves 3—5 times daily.

Intradermal-needle-embedding: Two of the main points and 1—2 of the supplementary points are selected according Syndrome Differentiation. After routine sterilization, subcutaneous needles are embedded in the selected points. With alternate use of the bilateral points, the treatment is given once every 3—5 days and 10 sessions constitute 1 therapeutic course with an interval of 7 days between courses. During treatment, ask the patients to press the stuck seeds themselves 3—5 times daily.

Remarks

(1) Auricular acupuncture proved to be effective for relieving tinnitus and deafness. However, since the cause is various, etiologic treatment is necessary for improving therapeutic effects.

(2) For deafness, auricular acupuncture is effective for patients with residual hearing but not satisfying for those with complete deafness.

Clinical reports

(1) Yang Yunkuan reported that auricular seed-pressing was effective for tinnitus and deafness. He selected Liver (MA—SC5), Kidney (MA—SC), Heart (MA—IC) and Subcortex (MA—AT1), Endocrine (MA—IC3) and Shenmen (MA—TF1) as main points. In case of dyspepsia, Spleen (MA—IC), Stomach (MA—IC) and Intestine (MA) were added. Two to three of the above points were used in each treatment with alternate use of the bilateral points. *Xi-*

ao Er Jing Feng Wan (Infantile Convulsion Pill) mixed with a little amount of *She Xiang* (Moschus) was used to press the selected points, which were renewed once every 7 days.

(2) Guan Zunxin et al reported 32 cases of tinnitus treated with auricular seed-pressing mainly at Internal Ear (MA–L), External Ear (MA–T), Liver (MA–SC5) and Subcortex (MA–AT1). Results: 12 cases were cured, 9 cases improved remarkably, 7 cases improved, and 4 cases were ineffective. The total effective rate was 87.5%.

32. Meniere's syndrome

Meniere's syndrome, also called membranous labyrinthine hydrops, is characterized clinically by recurrent episode of severe vertigo associated with deafness and tinnitus. It is encountered most often in men in the age group from 40–60, and 80% of the patients are initially affected on one ear, and then the other ear 2–3 years later. The cause is not known, but "endolymphatic hydrops" with marked dilatation of the cochlear duct is the pathologic finding. Meniere's disease may follow head trauma or middle ear infection, but many cases develop without apparent damage to the nervous system or ear.

Essentials of diagnosis

(1) Vertigo: Intermittent severe vertigo is the principal symptom. "Spinning" of surrounding objects is often noted. Nausea, vomiting and profuse perspiration are often associated. The attacks may last from a few minutes to several hours. The frequency of attacks varies considerably, even in the same patient. Patients may be absent from premonitory symptoms but some may have deafness, tinnitus, full sensation of the ear, nausea, etc. prior to onset.

(2) Tinnitus: Approximate 80% of the patients has tinnitus in varying degrees, which has a tendency of progressing along with repeated attacks.

(3) Decline of hearing: It is sensory, developing from low frequency to high frequency. The hearing loss is apt to be progressive, and is unilateral in 90% of cases.

(4) Nystagmus: It is a kind of horizontal and rotatory nystagmus and in direct proportion to vertigo in severity and time of lasting. Nystagmus may occur during attacks of vertigo.

Treatment

(1) Prescription (Fig. 4−32):

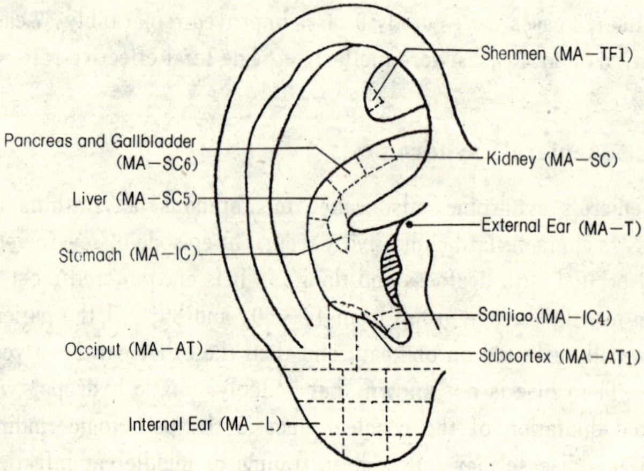

Fig. 4−32

Main points: Internal Ear (MA−L), Kidney (MA−SC), Shenmen (MA−TF1).

Supplementary points: Subcortex (MA−AT1), Liver (MA−SC5), Oancreas and Gallbladder (MA−SC6), Stomach (MA−IC), Sanjiao (MA−IC4), Occiput (MA−AT).

(2) Methods:

Needling with filiform needle: According to Syndrome Differentiation, 2−3 of the main points and 1−2 of the supplementary points are selected. After routine sterilization, the sensitive spots in the selected point loci are punctured bilaterally. The treatment can be given once daily, or twice daily for severe cases, with 10 sessions as a therapeutic course.

Intradermal-needle-embedding: Two to three of the main points and 1−2 of the supplementary points are selected according Syndrome Differentiation. After routine sterilization, subcutaneous needle is embedded in the selected points. For patients in acute stage, the treatment can be given at bilateral points once every 2—3 days; for patients in remission stage, the treatment can be given at unilateral points once every 3—5 days with alternate use of the bilateral points. Five treatments constitute 1 therapeutic course with an interval of 7 days between courses. During the period of treatment, ask the patients to press the embedded needles themselves 3—5 times daily.

Seed-pressing: All of the main points are used and 2—3 of the supplementary points are selected according Syndrome Differentiation. Magnetic pellet is the best choice, and vaccaria seed is applicable. With alternate use of the bilateral points, the treatment can be given once every 3—5 days and 5 sessions constitute 1 therapeutic course with an interval of 7 days between courses. During the period of treatment, ask the patients to press the stuck seeds themselves 3—5 times daily. This therapy is suitable for patient in the remission stage.

Drug-injection: The commonly-used drugs are vitamin B_1, vitamin B_{12}, *Dan Shen Zhu She Ye* (Radix Salviae Miltiorrhizae Injection) and*Huang Qi Zhu She Ye* (Radix Astragal Injection). In each treatment, 2—3 of the main points and 1—2 of the supplementary points are selected and each of them is injected 0.1—0.3 ml of drug solution. The treatment can be performed once daily and 10 times constitute 1 therapeutic course. Usually, points on the diseased side are initially treated, followed by the other side, alternating between them. In severe cases, bilateral points should be treated simultaneously.

Remarks

(1) Auricular acupuncture proved markedly effective for relieving symptoms of Meniere's syndrome. However, since many of these patients have a marked psychic overlay, reassurance is important.

(2) During the stage of attack, the patient should be advised to keep in bed quietly, to limit intake of salt and water and avoid smoking, alcoholic beverage, coffee and tea.

(3) If the patient suffers from frequent attacks, it is recommend-

ed to give the treatment in the remission stage.

Clinical reports

(1) Pan Jihua reported 68 cases of Meniere's syndrome treated with auricular seed-pressing therapy. Main points selected were Internal Ear (MA−L), Occiput (MA−AT), Liver (MA−SC5) and Kidney (MA−SC). In case of vomiting, Stomach (MA−IC), Sympathetic (MA−AH7) and Shenmen (MA−TF1) were added; and in case of severe dizziness and tinnitus, Sanjiao (MA−IC4), Shenmen (MA−TF1) and Temple (MA−AT) were added. With alternate use of the bilateral points, vaccaria seeds were used to press the selected points and they were changed once every other day. Five treatments constituted 1 therapeutic course. During the period of treatment, patients were asked to press the stuck points 5 times daily with each time lasting for 5 minutes. After 1−5 treatments, 61 cases were cured, 54 cases were improved, and 2 cases were ineffective. The total effective rate was 97%.

(2) Jia Zhenhua et al reported 20 cases of Meniere's syndrome treated with needling with filiform needles. Main points used were Occiput (MA−AT), Kidney (MA−SC), Central Rim (MA−AT) and Lesser Occiput (MA), supplemented with Internal Ear (MA−L), Ear Center (MA−H1), Cardia (MA−IC7), Pyloric (MA), Eye (MA−L1) and Spleen (MA−IC). Points were punctured with filiform needles. The four main points were needled first, and then 1−2 supplementary points which were selected according to different conditions. Needles were retained for 2−3 hours or 7−8 hours. Three days later, auricular seed-pressing was applied instead of needling to stabilize the therapeutic effects. Results: 16 cases recovered, three improved and one failed to respond. The total effective rate was 95%.

33. Toothache

Toothache is the most common symptom encountered in dental department. It can be caused by diseases of the tooth, periodontal tissues, jaw bone or nerves, such as dental caries, pulpitis, gingivitis, periodontal abscess and dentine hypersensitiveness. It may also be a reaction of a general disease.

Essentials of diagnosis

(1) Toothache, which is often aggravated by stimuli of cold, hot, sour and sweet.

(2) Examination may find dental cavity, percussion pain of the tooth, swelling and redness of the gum, and /or even discharge of pus.

Treatment

(1) Prescription (Fig. 4−33):

Main points: Jaw (MA−L), Anterior Ear lob (MA−L), Tooth (MA−L), Shenmen (MA−TF1).

Supplementary points: Subcortex (MA−AT1), Stomach (MA−IC), Kidney (MA−SC), Sanjiao (MA−IC4), Sympathetic (MA−AH7).

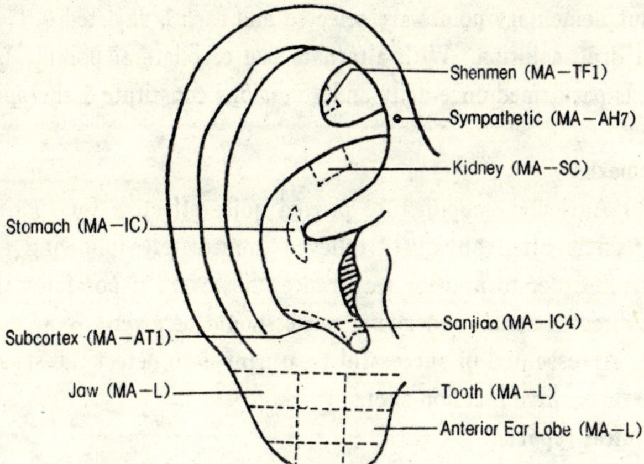

Fig. 4−33

(2) Methods:

Needling with filiform needles: Two to three of the main points and 1−2 of the supplementary points are selected according to Syndrome Differentiation. After routine sterilization, the selected points are punctured with filiform needles, which are retained for 20 − 30 minutes. For Excess type, needles are manipulated with strong stimulation techniques and the treatment is given 1—2 times daily; for Deficiency type, needles are manipulated with weak stimulation techniques and the treatment is given once daily or every other day. Four treatments constitute 1 therapeutic course.

Seed-pressing: All of the main points are used and 2—3 of the supplementary points are selected according Syndrome Differentiation. Magnetic pellet is the best choice, and vaccaria seed is applicable. With alternate use of the bilateral points, the treatment is given once every 3 days and 5 sessions constitute 1 therapeutic course with an interval of 7 days between courses. During the period of treatment, ask the patients to press the stuck seeds themselves 3—5 times daily. For severe pain, bilateral points should be treated simultaneously.

Drug-injection: Procaini hydrochloridum and penicillin are commonly used. In each treatment, 2—3 of the main points and 1—2 of the supplementary points are selected and each is injected 0.1—0.3 ml of drug solution. With alternate use of bilateral points, treatment is performed once daily and 4 sessions constitute 1 therapeutic course.

Remarks

(1) Auricular acupuncture proved quite effective for toothache and pain is often obviously relieved immediately following treatment. In order to prevent recurrence, however, if possible, treatment directed at the underlying cause should be given.

(2) An essential of successful treatment is to detect the sensitive spots or positive reaction spots.

Clinical reports

(1) Fang Luanhai reported that auricular seed-pressing therapy is rather good effective for toothache. He selected Tooth (MA—L), Anterior Ear Lob (MA—L), Shenmen (MA—TF1), Occiput (MA—AT) and other pain-sensitive spots. First detect the sensitive spots in the point locus, and then stick vaccaria seeds onto them with adhesive plaster. The treatment was given once every other day with alternate use of the bilateral points and the patients were asked to press the stuck seeds several times daily. Commonly,

toothache was relieved either partially or completely as soon as treatment was given and cured after 1—3 treatments.

(2) Zhou Li reported 30 cases of toothache treated with auricular acupuncture. Sanjiao (MA－IC4) was taken as main point and Shenmen (MA—TF1) as supplementary point. Method: first detect tenderness in the point locus, then puncture them with filiform needle after sterilization. The treatment was performed at the above points on the affected side once per day with four times constituting one course. For those who were afraid of needling, auricular seed-pressing with vaccaria seeds was applied instead and the patient was asked to press the stuck seeds until a hot sensation was produced 3—4 times daily. Four days constituted one therapeutic course. Of the 30 cases, 23 accepted needling and the remaining seven auricular seed-pressing. Results: in the needling group, after 1－4 treatments, 16 cases were cured, 6 were improved, and 1 were ineffective; in the auricular seed-pressing group, after one course of treatment (four days), 5 were cured and 2 were improved.

(3) Han Biying reported 72 cases of toothache treated by pressing the positive reaction spots with a probe. Method: on the interior side of antitragus, draw an equilateral triangle based on the line connecting Apex of Antitragus (MA－AT) and Central Rim (MA－AT). Detect a positive spot with a probe in the triangle, such as angioplerosis, patch aula or spot-like papula. Press the positive spot with a probe: first press it slightly for a while to produce a sharp stabbing pain, and then press heavily towards the rim of antitragus to produce an intolerable pain. Generally, the toothache will be relieved immediately. Results: 69 cases were cured, accounting for 95.85% of the total cases. Comparing with a routine acupuncture group (n=51 cases, cure rate was 78.51%), there was a significant difference ($P<0.05$) in favor of the auricular therapy.

34. Acute tonsillitis

Acute tonsillitis is a common diseases of the throat, frequently caused by infection of hemolytic streptococci, diplococcus pneumonia or staphylococci and clinically characterized by sudden onset with sort throat, fever, chills, headache, anorexia and malaise. Frequently, it occurs in winter or alteration of the season and affects children and juvenile.

Essentials of diagnosis

(1) The onset is sudden with obvious sore throat. The pain may radiate to the internal ear and be aggravated by swallowing.

(2) The tonsil is congestive and swollen, covered with yellowish white exudate which can be wiped away easily, and even multiple abscesses in severe cases.

(3) It may be accompanied with chill, fever, headache, mandibular lymphadenectasis, general discomfort.

(4) The white count may be elevated, and throat culture will show the infecting organism.

Treatment

(1) Prescription (Fig. 4—34):

Main points: Tonsil (MA—L), Adrenal Gland (MA—T).

Supplementary points: Lung (MA—IC1), Ear Apex (MA—H6), Stomach (MA—IC).

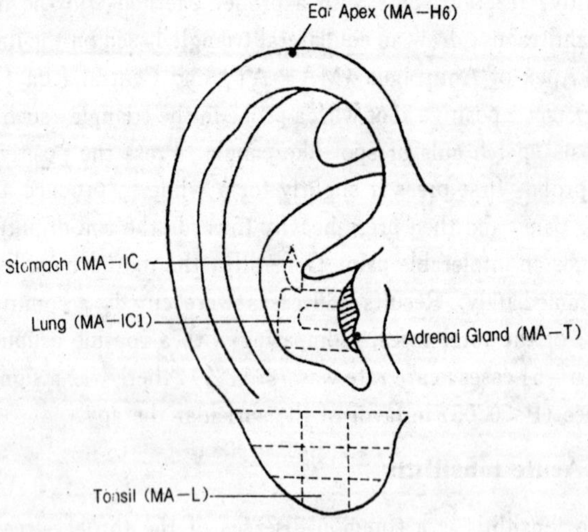

Fig. 4—34

(2) Methods:

Needling with filiform needle: All of the main points are used and 1－2 of the supplementary points are selected according Syndrome Differentiation. After detecting the sensitive spots in point loci and applying routine sterilization, the doctor punctures the points with filiform needles and retain them for 20－30 minutes. During retention, the needles are manipulated with a strong stimulation technique. The treatment can be given at bilateral points once daily and five sessions constitute one therapeutic course.

Bleeding therapy: One obvious vein in the upper part of the posterior auricular surface is selected in each treatment with alternate use of the two ears. After kneading or rubbing it to make it congestive and applying routine sterilization, the doctor pricks it with a three-edged needle to bleed 3－5 drops. The treatment can be given once daily and 4 times constitute 1 course with a 7 day interim between courses

Drug-injection: Procaini hydrochloridum and penicillin are commonly used. In each treatment, all of the main points and 1－2 of the supplementary points are selected and each is injected 0.2 ml of drug solution. With alternate use of bilateral points, the treatment is performed once daily and 4 sessions constitute 1 therapeutic course.

Intradermal-needle-embedding: In each treatment all of the main points are used and 1－2 of the supplementary points are selected according Syndrome Differentiation. Intradermal needles are embedded in the selected points and they are changed once every other day with 4 times as 1 therapeutic course.

Clinical reports

(1) According to clinical reports, bleeding therapy at veins of the posterior auricular surface is vary effective for acute tonsillitis.

(2) Li Yanwen reported 50 cases of acute tonsillitis treated with injection of penicillin at Tonsil (MA－L) (skin test of penicillin should be done before treatment). Treatment was given once daily with alternate use of the bilateral points. After treatment, 44 patients were cured, and 6 improved remarkably.

(3) Wang Jun et al reported 90 cases of acute tonsillitis treated

with pricking at Heat Point (MA). Heat Point (MA) is located in the area 0. 5 Cun inferior to Ear Apex (MA—H6). When performing treatment, prick the point with a three-edged needle and then squeeze it to bleed a little amount of blood. After treatment, all of the patients were cured, of which 35 cases were cured after 1 treatment, 24 after 2 treatments, and 3 after more than 3 treatments.

(4) A report of 25 cases of acute tonsillitis treated with auricular needling. Helix 6,4,3 (MA—H) were taken as main points and Helix 1,2,5 (MA—H) as supplementary points. In each treatment, two of the main points and one of the supplementary points were selected. Treatment was given once daily till the patient was cured. All of the patients were cured with a mean treatment of 3 times.

35. Acne vulgaris

Acne vulgaris is a common inflammatory disease of unknown cause that is apparently activated by androgens in those who are genetically predisposed. It may occur from puberty through the period of sex hormone activity. Eunuchs are spared. Similar involvement may occur in identical twins.

The disease is more common and more severe in males. Contrary to popular brief, it does not always clear spontaneously when maturity is reached. If untreated, it may persist into the fourth and even sixth decade of life.

Essentials of diagnosis

(1) Initially, comedo appears, which is the size of pinpoint. There are two types of comedo: white and black. The white type is characterized by white head and no cream white lipid droplets when it is squeezed with fingers. The black type is characterized by black head and lipid droplets when it is squeezed. If secondary infection occurs, comedo will turn into red papula eruption or small abscess.

(2) The skin lesions occur mainly over the face, neck, upper chest, back, and shoulders. Comedones are common.

(3) With slow course of illness, it is apt to recurrence. However, most patients can obtain reduction or recovery naturally after adolescent period.

(4) Generally, there are no subjective symptoms or only local itching and pain sensation.

Treatment

(1) Prescription (Fig. 4－35):

Main points: Ear Apex (MA－H6), Endocrine (MA－IC3), Lung (MA－IC1), Stomach (MA－IC).

Supplementary points: Adrenal Gland (MA－T), Shenmen (MA－TF1), Subcortex (MA－AT1), Heart (MA－IC), Cheek (MA－L), Large Intestine (MA－SC4).

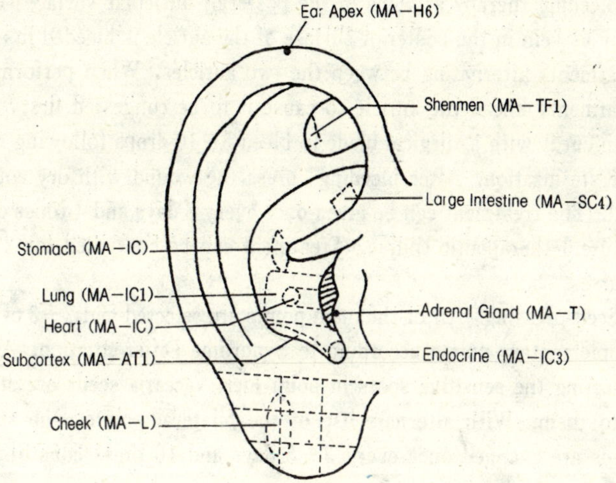

Fig. 4－35

(2) Methods:

Needling with filiform needle: Two to three of the main points and 1－2 of the supplementary points are selected according Syndrome Differentiation. After detecting the sensitive spots in point loci and applying routine sterilization, the doctor punctures them with filiform needles. The needles are retained for 30－45 minutes and manipulated with a rather strong stimulation technique every 5－10 minutes. The treatment is usually given at unilateral points once daily with alternate use of bilateral points and 10 sessions constitute 1 therapeutic course with a 10 day interim between courses.

Ear Apex (MA—H6) can be treated with bleeding therapy.

Bleeding therapy at auricular points: In each treatment 2 — 3 points are bleeded, alternating between the above points. When performing treatment, first knead the points to make them congestive, and then prick them with a three-edged needle or cut with a surgical blade to bleed naturally 1—2 drops for each point. After beddling, press the wound with dry cotton ball. The treatment can be done once every other day and 3 sessions constitute 1 therapeutic course with an interim of 5—7 days between courses.

Bleeding therapy at veins of the posterior auricular surface: One obvious vein in the posterior surface of the auricle is bleeded in each treatment, alternating between the two auricles. When performing treatment, knead the auricle to cause it to be congested first, and then cut it with a surgical blade to bleed 5—10 drops following routine sterilization. After bleeding, press the wound with dry cotton ball. The treatment can be given once every 3 days and 4 times constitute 1 therapeutic course. Treatment can be continued for 2—3 courses.

Seed-pressing: All of the main points are selected and 2—3 of the supplementary points according to Syndrome Differentiation. After detecting the sensitive spots in point loci, vaccaria seeds are stuck onto them. With alternate use of the bilateral points, the stuck seeds are changed once every 3—5 days and 10 times constitute 1 therapeutic course.

Remarks

(1) According to TCM, acne vulgaris is in most cases considered to be caused by Blood-Heat. Therefore, bleeding therapy can produce rather good effectiveness.

(2) During treatment, the patients should be advised to take light food, to give up smoking and drinking, to keep facial hygiene and to avoid exposure to oils and greases.

(3) To improve and stabilize therapeutic effects, aggravating or complicating emotional disturbances must be taken into consideration and treated appropriately.

Clinical reports

(1) Li Tong reported 14 cases of acne treated with auricular bleeding therapy. Main points used were Lung (MA－IC1), Endocrine (MA－IC3), Internal Genitals (MA－TF) and Cheek (MA－L) or Forehead (MA－AT), supplemented with Heart (MA－IC), Stomach (MA－IC), Subcortex (MA－AT1) and Adrenal Gland (MA－T). Select 2－3 main points and 3 supplementary points according to Syndrome Differentiation in each treatment. First knead the auricle mildly to make congestion, then cut an incision of 0.1－0.2 cm long in each point to bleed naturally. After bleeding, cover the wound with dry cotton ball. The treatment was given once daily with alternate use of bilateral points and 10 treatments constituted 1 therapeutic course.

(2) Liu Lianping reported 40 cases of acne treated with applying bleeding at veins of posterior surface of the auricle. Select one apparent vein in the posterior surface of the auricle, knead the auricle to cause congestive, and then cut it to bleed 5－10 drops following routine sterilization. After operation, press the wound with dry cotton ball to stop bleeding. If the first treatment failed to cure the disease, the second treatment was given 1 week later. After 1－3 treatment sessions, 18 patients recovered, 12 improved remarkably, 6 improved, and 4 failed to respond.

(3) Xu Yihong reported 80 cases of acne treated with auricular needling therapy. Main points used were Lung (MA－IC1) and Kidney (MA－SC). Supplementary points were added according to different symptoms: Spleen (MA－IC) for seborrhea, Large Intestine (MA－SC4) for constipation, Liver (MA－SC5) and Endocrine (MA－IC3) for dysmenorrhea, and points corresponding to the affected area for limited focus. Filiform needle of 15 mm long was used to puncture the selected points but the needle did not penetrate through the cartilage. The needles are retained for 15－30 minutes and manipulated 3－6 times during the period of needle retention. The treatment was given once every other day and 30 sessions constituted 1 therapeutic course. Results: 62 patients recovered, 11 improved remarkably, and 7 failed to respond. The total effective rate was 91.3%. The article pointed out that auricular acupuncture was

most effective for inflammatory acne, papula acne and pustular acne, second to which was severe acne. All the 7 cases of cystic acne and cachectic acne were ineffective.

Zhang Huanan reported 50 cases of acne treated with auricular seed-pressing therapy. Main points used were Lung (MA－IC1), Shenmen (MA－TF1), Sympathetic (MA－AH7) and Subcortex (MA－AT1). Vaccaria seeds were used for treatment with 5 treatment sessions constituting 1 course. Results: 12 cases were cured after 1 treatment course, 17 after 2 treatment courses, 13 after 3 treatment courses, and 5 after 4 treatment courses. The total cure rate was 94%. The remaining 3 cases were improved. A total effective rate of 100% was obtained.

36. Urticaria

Urticaria is an itching dermatosis, characterized mainly by wheal of the skin. It can result from many different stimuli, such as medicine, food and infection. The pathogenic mechanism may be either immunologic or nonimmunologic. The most common immunologic mechanism is the type Ⅰ hypersensitivity state mediated by IgE. Another immunologic mechanism involves the activation of the complement cascade, which produces anaphylatoxins. Those in turn can release histamine. Whether the pathogenesis is allergic or nonallergic, modulating factors affect mast cells and basophils to release mediators capable of producing urticaria lesions. These mediators include histamine, serotonin, kinins, leukotrienes, prostaglandins, acetylcholines, degradation products of fibrin, and anaphylatoxins that increase vascular permeability, producing wheals. Urticaria can affect people of all ages and both sexes.

Essentials of diagnosis

(1) Wheal, which presents abruptly. Initially, itching of the skin appears, later wheal presents. The wheal varies in size and form, accompanied with intolerable itching. The wheals may be fresh red, pink or pale in color, and the skin lesions appear paroxysmally without any trance left after disappearance. The skin lesions are indefinite, often disappearing from one place and appearing soon in anoth-

er place.

(2) Itching, which is severe and possibly accompanied with a sensation of hot or burning pain.

(3) Some patients may have fever (usually lower than 38 ℃), digestive symptoms such as nausea, vomiting, abdominal pain and diarrhea, and respiratory symptoms such as chest distress and dyspnea.

(4) Duration is varying. For acute uriticaria, it may recover after several days to two weeks. If urticaria attacks paroxysmally for over 1 month, it is considered as chronic one.

Treatment

(1) Prescription (Fig. 4—36):

Main points: Wind Stream (MA—SF), Adrenal Gland (MA—AT), Endocrine (MA—IC3), Lung (MA—IC1), Ear Apex (MA—H6).

Supplementary points: Liver (MA—SC5), Spleen (MA—IC), Large Intestine (MA—SC4), Small Intestine (MA—SC2), Shenmen (MA—AT1).

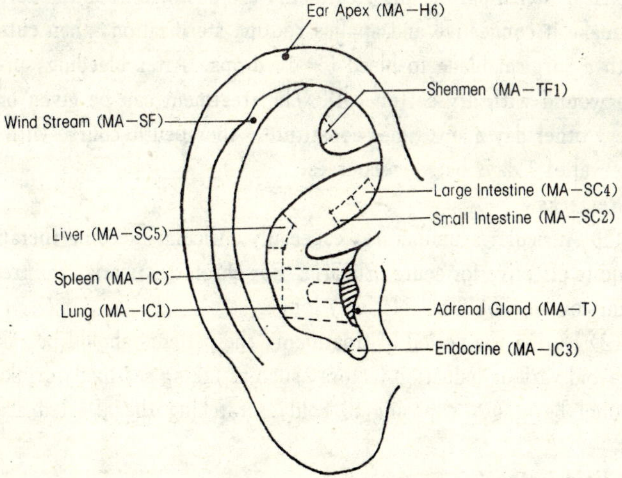

Fig. 4—36

(2) Methods:

Needling with filiform needle: Two to three of the main points and 1－2 of the supplementary points are selected according Syndrome Differentiation. First detect the sensitive spots in point loci, then puncture them with filiform needles following routine sterilization. The needles are retained for 30－45 minutes and manipulated with a rather strong stimulation technique every 5－10 minutes. The treatment can be given at unilateral points once daily with alternate use of bilateral points and 10 sessions constitute 1 therapeutic course with an interval of 10 days between courses. For chronic urticaria, the treatment can be given once every other day.

Seed-pressing: In each treatment, all of the main points and 2－3 of the supplementary points are selected, alternating between the two ears. After the sensitive spots are detected, vaccaria seed or magnetic pellet is stuck onto them. The stuck seeds change once every 3－5 days. During treatment, ask the patient to press the stuck seeds 5 times daily.

Bleeding therapy: In each treatment one apparent vein in the posterior surface of the auricle is selected with alternate use of the two auricles. When performing treatment, the doctor kneads the auricle to make it congestive and applies routine sterilization, then cuts it with a surgical blade to bleed 5－10 drops. After bleeding, press the wound with dry cotton ball. The treatment can be given once every other day and 2 times constitute 1 therapeutic course with an interval of 7 days between courses.

Remarks

(1) Auricular acupuncture, especially auricular bleeding therapy, is quite effective for acute urticaria. For chronic urticaria, the treatment course should be relatively longer.

(2) During the period of treatment, the patients should be asked to avoid various induction factors, such as taking sea food, drinking alcohol beverage, exposing to cold, scratching the affected area, etc.

Clinical reports

(1) Zhang Hehuan et al reported 42 cases of uritcaria treated with auricular needling. Points selected were: ① Lung (MA－IC1),

Small Intestine (MA－SC2) and Endocrine (MA－IC3); ② Heart (MA－IC), Large Intestine (MA－SC4) and Adrenal Gland (MA－T). The above two groups of points were used alternately. In addition, add Parotid Gland (MA) and Occiput (MA－AT) for cases with severe itching, and Wind Stream (MA－SF) or bleeding at posterior surface of the auricle for cases with slow response to treatment. Filiform needles of 15 mm long were used to puncture the selected points. The needles were retained for 30 minutes and manipulated every 10 minutes. The treatment was given once every other day. Intradermal-needle-embedding may be applied instead of needling, which was given once every 2－5 days with alternate use of the bilateral points. Results: 41 cases were cured, of which 9 were cured after 1 treatment, 24 after 2 treatments and 8 after 3 treatments, and 1 cases were ineffective. The total effective rate was 97%.

(2) Yi Zhenyun reported 25 cases of intractable urticaria treated with auricular seed-pressing, of which the shortest disease duration was 7 days while the longest 2 years. Points selected were: Lung (MA－IC1), Adrenal Gland (MA－T), Endocrine (MA－IC3), Shenmen (MA－TF1) and Wind Stream (MA－SF). Green gram and zinc oxide tape were used for pressing the points and the treatment was given once every 4 days. Results: 5, 8, 6, 3 and 3 cases were cured after 2, 3, 4, 6 and 7 treatments, respectively.

37. Flat wart

Flat wart is a kind of viral dermotoses, marked by benign neoplasm frequently affecting the face, dorsum of the hand and forearm. It is found mostly in young people, more in male than in female.

Essentials of diagnosis

(1) It often occurs abruptly as a papula eruption, first the size of needle-tip or a sesame seed, and later the size of a rice grain. The color is light brown or light grey, and the surface is smooth. They may appear either separately or densely.

(2) There is slight itching or no any obvious subjective symptom

in the diseased area.

(3) It may heal itself or recur again.

Treatment

(1) Prescription (Fig. 4—37):

Main points: Lung (MA—IC1), Adrenal Gland (MA—T), Points corresponding to the affected area.

Supplementary points: Ear Apex (MA—H6), Liver (MA—SC5), Spleen (MA—IC), Endocrine (MA—IC3).

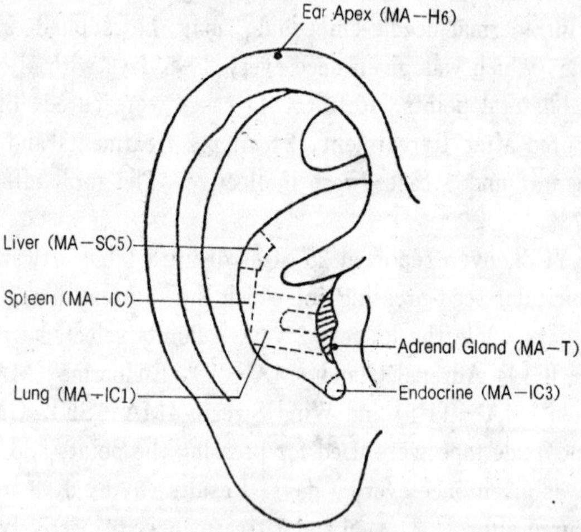

Fig. 4—37

(2) Methods:

Intradermal-needle-embedding: All of the main points are selected and 1—2 of the supplementary points are added according to Syndrome Differentiation. After routine sterilization, embed intradermal needles in the selected points. Commonly, one side of the points are used for each treatment with alternate use of the bilateral points. Needles are changed once every 2—3 days and 5 sessions constitute 1 therapeutic course.

Seed-pressing: All of the main points and 2—3 of the supplementary points are selected. After sensitive spots are detected, vaccaria seed or magnetic pellet is stuck onto them unilaterally with alternate use of the bilateral points and thay are changed once every 3－5 days. One therapeutic course consists of 7 treatments. During treatment, ask the patients to press the stuck seeds 5 times daily.

(3) Bleeding therapy: In each treatment one obvious vein in the upper or middle portion of the posterior auricular surface is selected with alternate use of the two auricles. When performing treatment, first knead the auricle to make it congestive and then cut it with a surgical knife blade to bleed 5－10 drops following routine sterilization. After operation, press the wound with dry cotton ball to stop bleeding followed by binding up with dressing. The treatment can be given once every 3 days and 4 treatments constitute 1 therapeutic course with an interval of 7 days between courses.

Remarks

(1) Auricular acupuncture produces rapid response for patients with short duration of illness while slow response for those with long duration.

(2) Appearance of a sudden increase of skin lesions with red surface and obvious itching sensation during the period of treatment indicates a tendency to recovery. Therefore, the treatment must be continued.

Clinical reports

(1) Zhao Qingyun reported 30 cases of flat wart treated with auricular seed-pressing. Main points selected were Lung (MA－IC1), Occiput (MA－AT), Endocrine (MA－IC3) and Adrenal Gland (MA－T), supplemented with points corresponding to the affected area. Vacaria seeds were used for treatment and the stuck seeds were changed once every 2－3 days with alternate use of the bilateral points. The patients were asked to press the points 3 times daily. Ten treatments constituted 1 therapeutic course. Results: 23 cases recovered, 2 cases improved markedly, and 5 cases failed to respond. The total effective rate was 83.4%.

(2) Zhang Shuxiao et al reported 41 cases of flat wart treated with auricular intradermal-needle-embedding therapy. Main points selected were Lung (MA－IC1), Endocrine (MA－IC3), Shenmen (MA－TF1) and Sympathetic (MA－AH7). When performing

treatment, first detect the sensitive spots in point loci with an electric detector, then embed thumbtack-like intradermal needle in them. Ten days of treatment was defined as a course and patients were asked to press the embedded needles several times daily. After 1—4 courses of treatment, a total effective rate of 95% was obtained.

(3) Li Qingzhi reported 34 cases of flat wart treated with bleeding therapy. Method: select one of the obvious capillary networks or shallow veins in the posterior surface of the auricle, and then prick it with a three-edged needle or cut it with a small surgical blade to bleed 5—10 drops followed by pressure on it with dry cotton ball to stop bleeding. Of the 34 cases, 22 cases were cured after 1—3 treatments, 10 cases were cured after 4—6 treatments, 1 case was improved remarkably, and 1 case was improved mildly.

(4) Qiu Zaijing reported 102 cases of youth wart treated with intradermal-needle-embedding. Lung (MA—IC1), Stomach (MA—IC) and Subcortex (MA—AT1) were selected as the main points, supplemented with the points corresponding to the affected area. The needles were changed once every 3 days with alternate use of the two ears. Results: cured in 75 cases, marked by disappearance of all warts after 3—6 treatment sessions; improved in 17 cases, marked by partial disappearance of warts after 7—10 treatment sessions; and failed to respond in 10 cases. The total effective rate was 90%.

38. Chloasma

Chloasma is a kind of skin disease, characterized by facial pigment hyperplasia. It can be seen in both men and women, but more frequently in women with pregnancy or irregular menstruation. The cause of the disease remains unknown. Some patients develop it following chronic diseases, such as hepatic disorders, tuberculosis and chronic alcoholism, and some following long-term administration of drugs, such as chorpromazini hypdrochloridum and phenytoinum natricum (dilation).

Essentials of diagnosis

(1) Skin lesions are usually found on the face, neck, nose, or around the mouth, which are often distributed symmetrically and in butterfly-form.

(2) Skin lesions show yellowish brown or dark brown with a boundary being either clear or indistinct. The patches vary in size, which may emerge into each other forming a large patch, and the surface of the patches is smooth. The condition can be aggravated by too much exposure to sun-light.

(3) The course of the disease is protracted, and the patients have no local subjective discomfort. A few patients may recover naturally.

Treatment

(1) Prescription (Fig. 4—38):

Main points: Points corresponding to the affected area, Liver (MA—SC5), Lung (MA—IC1), Endocrine (MA—IC3).

Supplementary points: Internal Genitals (Ma—TF), Kidney (NA—SC), Adrenal Gland (MA—T).

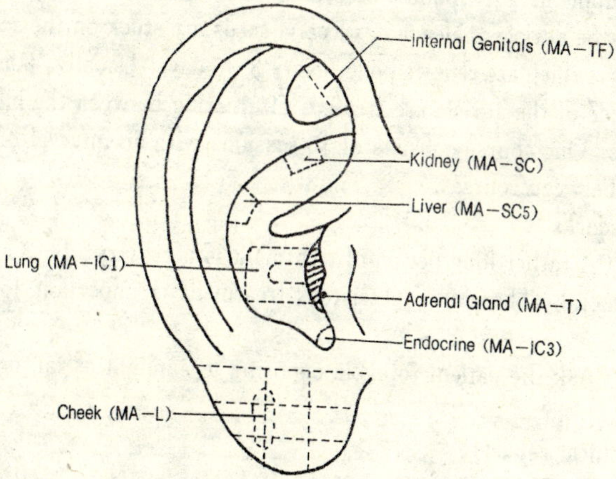

Fig. 4—38

(2) Methods:

Bleeding therapy: Two to three of the main points and 1—2 of the supplementary points are selected according Syndrome Differentiation. After routine sterilization, the doctor cuts an incision of 3—5 mm long or of cross-form in each selected point to cause oozing of blood, followed by pressing on it with sterilized dry cotton ball to stop bleeding. Usually, one side of the auricle is treated in each treatment, alternating with the other side of the auricle at intervals of 2—3 days. One therapeutic course consists of 4 sessions with an interval of 10 days between 2 courses.

Needling with filiform needle: According to Syndrome Differentiation, 2—3 of the main points and 2—3 of the supplementary points are selected for each treatment. After detecting the sensitive spots, points are punctured with filiform needles following routine sterilization. The needles are retained for 20—30 minutes. With alternate us of the bilateral points, treatment is given once daily or every other day and 10 sessions constitute 1 course with an interval of 10 days between courses.

(3) Seed-pressing: All of the main points are selected and 2—3 of the supplementary points according to Syndrome Differentiation. After the auricle is cleaned, vaccaria seeds are stuck on the selected points, which are renewed once every 3—5 days. Usually, points on one side of the auricle are treated, alternating between the bilateral points. One course consists of 10 sessions with an interval of 5—7 days between courses.

Remarks

(1) A rather long period of treatment is necessary, 1—3 months in general. Therefore, persistent treatment is important for success.

(2) Ask the patient to avoid exposing to sunlight as far as possible.

Clinical reports

(1) Du Wei et al reported 50 cases of chloasma treated with auricular seed-pressing. Main points used were Shenmen (MA—TF1), Internal genitals (MA—TF), Kidney (MA—SC), Liver (MA—SC5), Spleen (MA—IC), Endocrine (MA—IC3) and Subcortex (MA—AT1), supplemented with Large Intestine (MA—SC4),

Stomach (MA—IC), Ovary (MA), Heart (MA—IC) and Gallbladder (MA—SC6). Treatment was given once every other day and 15 sessions constituted 1 course. After 3 courses of treatment. 26 cases were cured, 15 cases improved, 7 cases mildly improved, and 2 cases failed to respond. The total effective rate was 96%.

(2) Xue Wei reported 200 cases of chloasma treated with auricular seed-pressing. Cheek (MA—L) was selected as the main point, supplemented with Upper Lung (MA), Lower Lung (MA), External Nose (MA—T1), and Large Intestine (MA—SC4). Treatment was given once every other day and 15 sessions constituted 1 course. Results: 120 cases were cured, 72 cases improved remarkably, and 8 cases were ineffective. The total effective rate was 96%.

(3) Xia Yuqing reported 183 cases of chloasma treated with auricular bleeding therapy. Main point selected were Heat Point (MA), Boil (MA) and Subcortex (MA—AT1), supplemented with Endocrine (MA—IC3), Spleen (MA—IC) or Stomach (MA—IC). A surgical knife blade was used to cut the selected point 0.1 cm in depth. After cutting, clean the point with alcohol cotton ball, and then press it with dry cotton ball to stop bleeding. In each treatment only one of the above points was treated. The treatment was given nce every other day and 15 sessions constituted 1 course with an interval of 7—10 days between courses. The treatment can be continued for successive 2—3 courses. Results: 120 cases were cured, 72 cases improved remarkably, and 8 cases were not improved. The total effective rate was 96%.

39. Withdrawal from smoking

Smoking has all harm but good. A long history of smoking produces harm to various system and organs, such as the respiratory system, the cardiovascular system, the gastrointestinal system, the nervous system, the liver and the kidney, and increase the danger of developing cancer, coronary heart disease, pulmonary heart disease, gastroduodenal ulcer, chronic bronchitis, etc. It is reported that Seventy-five thousand people die of lung cancer in the USA annually, and almost all of these deaths are due to smoking or exposure to secondary tobacco smoke. Smoking is even more dangerous for women as it can elicit irregular menstruation, abortion, premature labor, affect the development of fetus, and even lead to fetal malformation. Smokers often suffer from various discomfort when they try to give it up, such as restlessness, lack of concentration, lassitude, dizziness, headache, irritability and vomiting.

Treatment

(1) Prescription (Fig. 4—39):

Main points: Lung (MA—IC1), Shenmen (MA—TF1), Subcortex (MA—AT1).

Supplementary points: Stomach (MA—IC), Mouth (MA—IC5), Heart (MA—IC), Adrenal Gland (MA—T), Endocrine (MA—IC3).

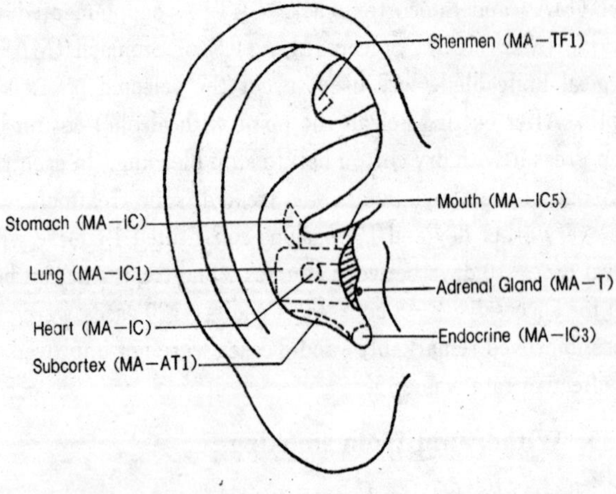

Fig. 4—39

(2) Methods:

Needling with filiform needle: All of the main points are selected and 2—3 of the supplementary points according Syndrome Differentiation. Filiform needles of 15 mm long are used to puncture the selected points following routine sterilization. The needles are retained for 20—30 minutes and manipulated 2—3 times during retention of needle. The reatment is given once daily or every other day with alternate use of the bilateral points. If bilateral points are treated simultaneously, points can be classified into two groups, alternating between them.

Intradermal-needle-embedding: In each treatment 2—3 of the main points and 1—2 of the supplementary points are selected. If a group of points are described, they can be treated unilaterally, alternating between the bilateral points. If two groups of points are prescribed, they can be treated bilaterally, alternating between the two groups. Needles are changed once every 3—5 days and the smokers are asked to press the treated points 3—5 time daily.

Auricular electroacupuncture: With alternate use of the above points, two points, one main point and one supplementary, are selected in each treatment and treated bilaterally. Commonly, the main point is connected to the positive electrode while the supplementary point to the negative electrode. Points are stimulated with dense-disperse wave for 30—40 minutes. The treatment an be given once daily and ten sessions constitute one course.

Remarks

(1) Auricular acupuncture is considered as one of the most satisfactory therapies for cessation of smoking as it is simple, highly effective and quickly responsive.

(2) The efficacy of auricular acupuncture in cessation of smoking is often temporary. Therefore, whether a smoker can finally give it up or not is dependent on his willpower.

Clinical reports

(1) Li Bening reported 27 smokers who accepted auricular intradermal-needle-embedding therapy for cessation of smoking. A total of short-term effective rate of 85% was obtained. Points selected were Lung (MA—IC1), Stomach (MA—IC) and Shenmen (MA—TF1). When performing treatment, detect sensitive spots in point loci first, and then embed intradermal needle in them accurately following routine sterilization. Needles were fixed with adhesive plaster and retained for 5—6 days. During the period of needle retention, the smokers were asked to press the treated points 3—5 times daily, especially when they developed a desire for cigarette.

(2) Fang Youan et al reported that auricular acupuncture can markedly lower smoker's taste threshold values of sweat and sour. Plasma cortisol content, which was higher in smokers than that in non-smokers ($P<0.05$), lowered to levels slightly below basal value after auricular acupuncture treatment.

(3) Ju Xianshui reported 80 smokers who accepted auricular electroacupuncture therapy, of which 24 were females. The history of smoking ranged from one year to 40 years with the mean daily consumption of 36 cigarettes, and 42.5% of the smokers had a smoking history of over 15 years. Shenmen (MA-TF1) and Stopping Smoking Area1 (MA) which was located as the most sensitive spot between Lung (MA-IC3) and Trachea (MA-IC2) were selected and stimulated with auricular electroacupuncture 30 minutes for each treatment. Treatment was given once every other day. After 1-3 treatments, 38 cases were improved remarkably, marked by complete cessation of smoking; 22 cases were improved, marked by smoking being reduced to less than 5 cigarettes daily; and 9 cases were mildly improved.

(4) Chen Xiuzhen et al reported 63 smokers who accepted auricular electroacupuncture therapy in combination auricular seed-pressing therapy for giving up smoking. Points used were Shenmen (MA-TF1), Lung (MA-IC1), Subcortex (MA-AT1) and Adrenal Gland (MA-T). First detect tender spots in the point area, then puncture them with filiform needles of NO. 30 and 1 inch long to produce a sensation of distending pain or burning after sterilization. Shenmen (MA-TF1) and Lung (MA-IC1) were connected to an electrical stimulator. The successive wave of 200 Hz was selected and the output intensity was increased gradually to the patient's maximal tolerance. Needles were retained for 30 minutes. After withdrawal of the needles, auricular seed-pressing with vaccaria seeds was applied to Shenmen (MA-TF1) and Lung (MA-IC1) on the opposite ear. Ask the patient to press the stuck seeds several times to enhance stimulation, especially when a smoking desire presented. The treatment was performed once per day with seven treatments constituting one therapeutic course. Results: remarkably ef-

fective obtained in 25 cases (39. 68%), marked by withdrawal of smoking; mildly effective in 22 cases (34. 92%), marked by smoking being reduced to 4—7 cigarettes daily; and ineffective in 9 cases (14. 29%).

40. Simple obesity

Obesity refers to excessive fat accumulated in the body. It can be classified as simple and secondary types. Generally called obesity denotes the simple type, which is defined as 20% over the standard weight.

The standard body weight can be calculated with the following formulas:

For those taller than 150 cm:

Standard weight (kg) = [height(cm) − 100] × 0. 9.

For those shorter than 150 cm:

Standard weight (kg) = height(cm) − 100.

Although obesity is common presenting "endocrine" complaint, the overwhelming majority of cases are due to excessive food intake or physical inactivity, or both. There is some experimental evidence favoring the concept that there are different rates of thermogenesis in obese and nonobese individuals, but the matter remains controversial. It is clear, however, that the obesity is always the result of a positive energy balance and will not occur if "excess" calories are not ingested.

Obesity may occur in people at any age, but more common in middle-aged females.

Essentials of diagnosis

(1) Body weight exceeds standard weight by over twenty per cent.

(2) Simple obesity is usually asymptomatic. In severe cases, however, it may be accompanied with such symptoms as dizziness, headache, fatigue, a tendency to perspiration, emotional depression, abdominal distention, hypogonadism, etc.

(3) Those resulting from nervous, endocrine or metabolic diseases and excessive muscles are excluded.

Treatment

(1) Prescription (Fig. 4—40):

Main points: Stomach (MA—IC), Mouth (MA—IC5), Hunger Point (MA), Spleen (MA—IC), Endocrine (MA—IC3).

Supplementary points: Shenmen (MA—TF1), Subcortex (MA—AT1), Kidney (MA—SC), Sanjiao (MA—IC4), Large Intestine (MA—SC4), Small Intestine (MA—SC2).

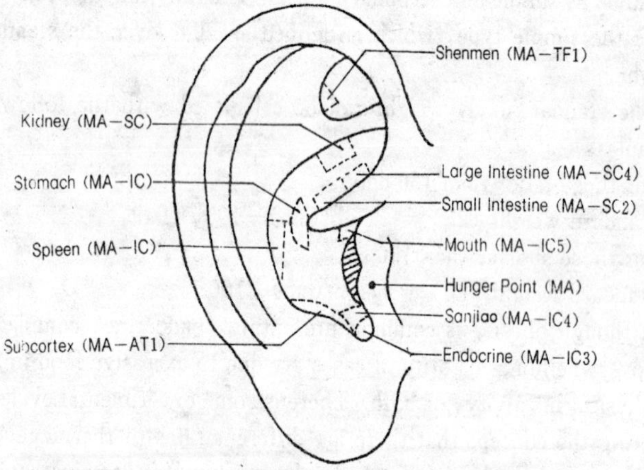

Fig. 4—40

(2) Methods:

Seed-pressing: All of the main points are used and 2—3 of the supplementary points are added according to Syndrome Differentiation. The sensitive spots in point loci are detected first, and then vaccaria seeds are stuck on them after they are cleaned with alcohol cotton ball. Points on one side are treated for each treatment, alternated with points on the other side. The stuck seeds are changed once every 3—5 days and 10 sessions constitute 1 course with an interval of 5—7 days between courses. Ask the patients to press the treated points 3—5 times daily, especially before meal and when they feel hungry.

Intradermal-needle-embedding: Two to three of the main points and 1—2 of the supplementary points are selected according to Syndrome Differentiation. After routine sterilization, intradermal needles are embedded in the selected points and they are changed once every 3—5 days. During retention of needles, ask the patients to press the treated points 20 times for each point before each meal. Points on one side are treated in each treatment, alternated with points on the other side. One course consists of 10 treatments with an interval of 10 days between courses.

Drug-injection: Two to three of the main points and 1—2 of the supplementary points are selected according to Syndrome Differentiation. After routine sterilization, each point is injected 0.1—0.3 ml of 2% procaine injection. The treatment can be performed at bilateral points once every 3—5 days and 10 sessions constitute 1 course.

Remarks

(1) Auricular acupuncture is effective for simple obesity, it, however, is not suitable for hereditary one. Clinical observation shows that most patients can obtain 1—3 kg weight loss after 1—2 treatment courses. The weight may not reduce or ever increase during the following period of successive treatments. However, if the treatment is continued, the weight may reduce gradually again. Therefore, persistent treatment is important for successful treatment.

(2) The patient can perform self-treatment of massage or finger-pressing on relevant auricular points to stabilize therapeutic effects.

(3) The patient should be advised to be moderate in eating and to avoid taking food rich in carbohydrate.

(4) Exercise can increase consumption of caloricity. Therefore, the patients should be encouraged to do more exercise.

Clinical reports

(1) Zhang Zhongzhi reported 110 cases of obesity treated with auricular needling. Large Intestine (MA—SC4), Small Intestine (MA—SC2) and Endocrine (MA—IC3) were selected and subcutaneous needles were embedded in them. Needles were changed once every 3 days and 10 sessions constituted 1 course. After 3 courses of treatment, the mean body weight of 71.9±10.8 kg was reduced to 67.4±10.04 kg, showing a significant difference before and after treat-

ment (P<0. 05).

(2) Xu Youqiang et al reported 96 cases of obesity treated with auricular seed—pressing. Main points selected were Hunger Point (MA), Shenmen(MA—TF1), Stomach(MA—IC), Cardia(MA—IC7), Esophagus (MA—IC6) and Abdomen Point (MA). Supplementary points were added according to accompanying symptoms: Thirst Point (MA) for excessive appetite and a tendency to thirst, Large Intestine (MA—SC4) for constipation, and Groove of Posterior Surface (MA—PS) for hypertension. First determine the sensitive spot in the point locus with an auricular detector, and then stick vaccaria seeds on them. With alternate use of the bilateral points, Treatment was given at points on one side of the auricle in each treatment and 6 sessions instituted 1 course. During the period of treatment, ask the patients to press the stuck seeds no less than 5 times daily with 20 seconds for each point until a local sensation of soreness, distention or hot was produced. After 3 sources of treatment, 93 cases obtained weight loss of 0. 5—11. 5 kg, 2 cases remained unchanged, and 1 case got weigh gain. Among the 96 cases, 37 cases had hyperlipemia, of which, after 3 months of treatment, 7 cases had cholesterol restored to normal value, 12 cases had triglyceride restored to normal value, and 8 cases had high density lipoprotein (HDL) and low density lipoprotein (HDL) restored to normal value.

(3) Lu Zhenchu et al reported 29 cases of obesity treated with auricular seed-pressing. Points used were Shenmen (MA — TF1), Stomach (MA — IC), Lung (MA — IC3) and Endocrine (MA — IC3). Patients were asked to press the stuck seeds before each meal with each times lasting for 10 minutes. After 1 course of treatment (10 sessions), triglyceride lowered in 19 cases with a mean drop of (18. 63 mg), cholesterol lowered in 18 cases with a mean drop of 12. 64 kg, high density lipoprotein (HDL) raised in 16 cases, and low density lipoprotein (HDL) raised in 16 cases. Statistic analysis showed there was a significant difference of the LDL before and after treatment (P>0. 01), but there was no significant difference of others.

(4) Cui Shugui reported 1015 cases of obesity treated with auricular intradermal-needle-embedding therapy. Main points used were Large Intestine (MA—SC4), Stomach (MA—IC), Sanjiao (MA—IC4), Endocrine (MA—IC3) and Shenmen (MA—TF1). Embedding of subcutaneous needles therapy was applied once every 3—5 days with 5 treatment sessions constituting 1 therapeutic course. Results: marked effect obtained in 264 cases (26%), manifested by weight loss of over 5 kg; mild effect in 370 cases (36.5%), manifested by weight loss of 3—5 kg; no effect in 381 cases (37.5%). The total effective rate was 62.5%.

Appendix

Ⅰ. Standard Auricular Points accepted by WHO Regional Officer for the Western Pacific in 1987

1. Points with alphanumeric coding

Chinese Pinyin	English nomenclature	Coding
Erzhong	Ear Center	MA—H1
Zhi Chang	Rectum	MA—H2
Niaodao	Urethra	MA—H3
Waishengzhiqi	External Genitals	MA—H4
Gangmen	Anus	MA—H5
Erjian	Ear Apex	MA—H6
Zhi	Fingers	MA—SF1
Wan	Wrist	MA—SF2
Zhou	Elbow	MA—SF3
Jian	Shoulder	MA—SF4
Suogu	Clavicle	MA—SF5
Gen	Heel	MA—AH1
Huai	Ankle	MA—AH2
Xi	Knee	MA—AH3
kuan	Hip	MA—AH4
Tun	Buttocks	MA—AH5
Zuogushenjing	Sciatic Nerve	MA—AH6
Jiaogan	Sympathetic	MA—AH7
Jingzhui	Cervical Vertebrae	MA—AH8
Xiongzhi	Thoracic Vertebrae	MA—AH9
Jing	Neck	MA—AH10
Xiong	Chest	MA—AH11
Shenmen	Ear Shenmen	MA—TF1
Waibi	External Nose	MA—T1
Pingjian	Apex of Tragus	MA—T2
Yanhou	Pharynx and Larynx	MA—T3
Pizhixia	Subcortex	MA—AT1
Fei	Lung	MA—IC1
Qiguan	Trachea	MA—IC2

Chinese Pinyin	English nomenclature	Coding
Neifenmi	Endocrine	MA—IC3
Sanjiao	Triple Energy	MA—IC4
Kou	M outh	MA—IC5
Shidao	Esophagus	MA—IC6
Penmen	Cardia	MA—IC7
Shierzhichang	Duodenum	MA—SC1
Xiaochang	Small Intestine	MA—SC2
Lanwei	Appendix	MA—SC3
Dachang	Large Intestine	MA—SC4
Gan	Liver	MA—SC5
Yidan	Pancreas and Gallbladder	MA—SC6
Shuniaoguan	Ureter	MA—SC7
Pangguang	Bladder	MA—SC8
Yan	Eye	MA—L1

2. Auricular points without alphanumeric coding

Chinese Pingyin	English nomenclature	Coding
Fengxi	Wind Stream	MA—ST
Zhi	Toe	MA—AH
Yaodizhui	Lumbosacral	MA—AH
Fu	Abdomen	MA—AH
Penqiang	Pelvis	MA—TF
Jiaowozhong	Meddle Triangular Fossa	MA—TF
Neishengzhiqi	Internal Genitals	MA—TF
Jiaowoshang	Superior Triangular Fossa	MA—TF
Shenshangxian	Adrenal Gland	MA—T
Duipingjian	Apex of Antitragus	MA—AT
Yuanzhong	Central Rim	MA—AT
Zhen	Occiput	MA—AT
Nie	Temple	MA—AT
E	Forehead	MA—AT
Xin	Heart	MA—IC
Pi	Spleen	MA—IC
Wei	Stomach	MA—IC
Shen	Kidney	MA—SC

Chinese Pingyin	English nomenclature	Coding
Tingjiao	Angle of Superior Concha	MA—SC
Ya	Tooth	MA—L
She	Tongue	MA—L
He	Jaw	MA—L
Chuiqian	Anterior Ear lobe	MA—L
Mu1	Eye1	MA—L
Neier	Internal Ear	MA—L
Mianjia	Cheek	MA—L
Biantaoti	Tonsil	MA—L
Shangergen	Upper Ear Root	MA—PS
Ermigen	Root of Vagus	MA—PS
Xiaergen Lower	Ear root	MA—PS
Erbeigou	Groove of Posterior Surface	MA—PS
Erbeixin	Heart of Posterior Surface	MA—PS
Erbeipi	Spleen of Posterior Surface	MA—PS
Erbeigan	Liver of Posterior Surface	MA—PS
Erbeifei	Lung of Posterior Surface	MA—PS
Erbeishen	Kidney of Posterior Surface	MA—PS

Ⅱ. Auricular Points Adopted by China Association of Acup u ntureand Moxibustion in 1987

Apart from the above 79 points, the following 11 points are in cluded.

Chinese Pinyin	English nomenclature	Coding
Ganyang	Liver Yang	MA—H
Lun1	Helix1	MA—H
Lun2	Helix2	MA—H
Lun3	Helix3	MA—H
Lun4	Helix4	MA—H
Lun5	Helix5	MA—H
Lun6	Helix6	MA—H
Waier	External Ear	MA—T
Neibi	Internal Nose	MA—T
Tingzhong	Middle of Superior Concha	MA—SC
Mu2	Eye2 Concha	MA—L
Mu2	Eye2	MA—L

耳针疗法

肖　飞
魏履霜　著
肖　飞
荆　蓁　译

*

山东科学技术出版社出版
济南市玉函路 16 号　邮政编码　250002
中国山东莱芜市印刷厂印刷
中国国际图书贸易总公司发行
中国北京车公庄西路 35 号
北京邮政信箱第 399 号　邮政编码　100044

*

1996 年(大 32)　1 版 1 次
ISBN 7-5331-1835-9
R·530
07200
14-E-3025P